GENETIC ASPECTS OF
HOST-PARASITE RELATIONSHIPS

SYMPOSIA OF THE
BRITISH SOCIETY FOR PARASITOLOGY
VOLUME 14

GENETIC ASPECTS OF
HOST-PARASITE RELATIONSHIPS

EDITED BY

ANGELA E. R. TAYLOR

AND

R. MULLER

London School of Hygiene and
Tropical Medicine
Keppel Street, London WC1E 7HT

BLACKWELL SCIENTIFIC PUBLICATIONS

OXFORD LONDON EDINBURGH MELBOURNE

© 1976 by Blackwell Scientific Publications
Osney Mead, Oxford, England
8 John Street, London WC1, England
9 Forrest Road, Edinburgh, Scotland
P.O. Box 9, North Balwyn, Victoria, Australia

ISBN

First published 1976

British Library Cataloguing in Publications Data
Genetic aspects of host-parasite relationships —
    (British Society for Parasitology. Symposia;
    vol. 14). Bibl. — Index
    ISBN 0-632-00099-6
    1. Taylor, Angela Elizabeth Russell
    2. Muller, Ralph
    3. Series
    574.5'24 QH547
    Host-parasite relationships-Congresses.
    Genetics-Congresses.

Distributed in the U.S.A. by
J. B. Lippincott Company, Philadelphia
and in Canada by
J. B. Lippincott Company of Canada Ltd,
Toronto

Printed in Great Britain

CONTENTS

PREFACE   vii

MOSQUITO GENETICS IN RELATION TO
FILARIAL INFECTIONS   1
W. W. Macdonald

GENETIC FACTORS IN RODENT MALARIA
PARASITES AND THEIR EFFECT ON HOST-
PARASITE RELATIONSHIPS   25
D. Walliker

GENETICS OF THE HOST-PARASITE
RELATIONSHIP BETWEEN *BIOMPHALARIA
GLABRATA* AND *SCHISTOSOMA MANSONI*   45
C. S. Richards

HYBRIDIZATION OF SCHISTOSOMES AND
SOME OF ITS IMPLICATIONS   55
C. A. Wright and V. Southgate

THE ECOLOGICAL GENETICS OF HOST-
PARASITE RELATIONSHIPS   87
B. C. Clarke

SUBJECT INDEX   105

AUTHOR INDEX   108

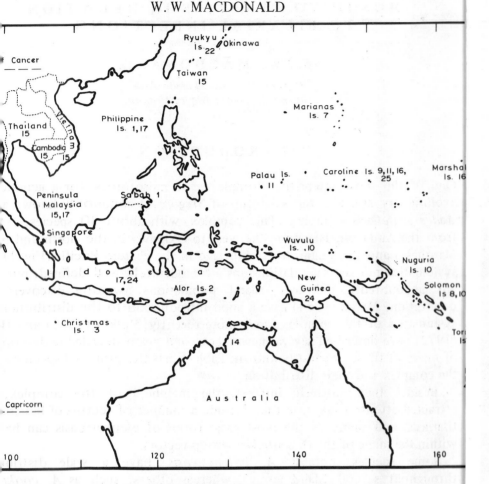

Fig. 1. The geographical distribution of the *Aedes (Stegomyia) scutellaris* mosquito complex. The list of species corresponding to the numbers on the map are given in Table 1.

mpatibility may occur in both parental crosses or only in one. Such rectional and unidirectional incompatibility has often been compared the situation in the *Culex pipiens* complex, in which incompatibility ween strains has been utilized for genetic control experiments. The nd consideration concerns the genetic basis of susceptibility in the quitoes to infection with filariae. If a single gene controls susceptibility in the *A. scutellaris* complex, as is the case with *A. aegypti*, it may be ible to construct a replacement population which would have most of genome of one of the vector species but which would differ by being refractory to infection and incompatible in both directions, or almost with the vector.

his review summarizes present knowledge of the relationships within the

MOSQUITO GENETICS IN RI
TO FILARIAL INFECTI

W. W. MACDONALD

Department of Medical Entomology,
Liverpool School of Tropical Medicine

INTRODUCTION

One of the most interesting complexes of mosqui
evolutionary study is the subgroup of *Stegomyia* co
Aedes scutellaris complex. This complex, with abo
from the Andaman Islands in the west to Okinawa i
Marquesas and the Tuamotu Archipelago in the east
systematics and species relationships are moderately
are undoubtedly unknown island populations a
description. Marks (1954) gave a good introduction
systematics of the complex, and, more recently, Be
(1972) have described several new species and given
of many of those previously known. Table 1 lists the
the complex and their distribution.

Besides their intrinsic interest, the members
attracted attention because they include a number c
filariasis, and many of the most gross forms of el
within the range of the *A. scutellaris* group vectors.

Some species, notably *A. polynesiensis*, hav
throughout several island groups, whereas others,
known only from one island. Such a distributio
populations well separated by natural barriers, migh
vector populations may not be too difficult. How
range of natural and artificial larval habitats which a
larval control by chemicals is usually not practical, a
the adults make control of adult populations expens

In theory, island populations might be suppresse
genetic control techniques and the *A. scutellaris*
quoted as a group which merits study with th
considerations have given support to this proposal
interspecific crossing relationships. Some species
almost fully fertile, whereas others, although they
readily with one another, produce eggs whic

1

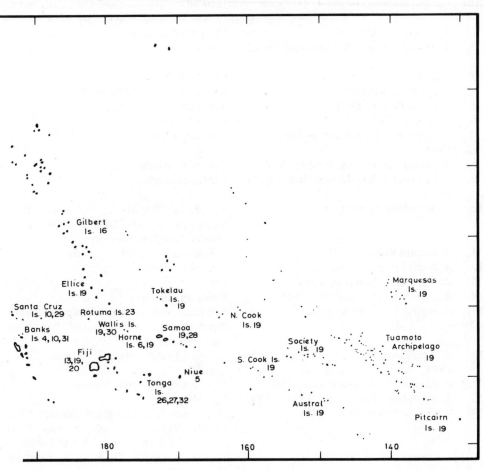

A. *scutellaris* complex together with those aspects of the genetics of other mosquitoes, especially *C. pipiens*, which are relevant to the long-term aim of genetic control of a filariasis vector population.

HYBRIDIZATION EXPERIMENTS

The members of the *A. scutellaris* complex can be fairly easily colonized in the laboratory, but because of their geographical isolation many species are difficult to collect and correspondingly few hybridization experiments have been carried out. However, those interspecific crosses that have been made have given most interesting results. In discussing them it is worth bearing in

Table 1

The principal members of the *Aedes* (*Stegomyia*) *scutellaris* complex and their distribution

1.	*A. alcasidi* Huang, 1972	Philippines, Sabah
2.	*A. alorensis* Bonne-Wepster and Brug, 1932	Alor Island
3.	*A. andrewsi* Edwards, 1926	Christmas Island
4.	*A. aobae* Belkin, 1962	Banks Islands, New Hebrides
5.	*A. cooki* Belkin, 1962	Niue Island
6.	*A. futunae* Belkin, 1962	Horne Islands
7.	*A. guamensis* Farner and Bohart, 1944	Marianas Islands
8.	*A. gurneyi* Stone and Bohart, 1944	Solomon Islands
9.	*A. hakanssoni* Knight and Hurlbut, 1949	Caroline Islands
10.	*A. hebrideus* Edwards, 1926	Wuvulu Is., Nuguria Is., Solomon Islands, Santa Cruz Islands, Torres Islands, Banks Islands, New Hebrides
11.	*A. hensilli* Farner, 1945	Caroline Islands, Palau Islands
12.	*A. hoguei* Belkin, 1962	Solomon Islands
13.	*A. horrescens* Edwards, 1935	Fiji
14.	*A. katherinensis* Woodhill, 1949	Northern Australia
15.	*A. malayensis* Colless, 1962	Andaman and Nicobar Islands, Singapore, Peninsular Malaysia, Thailand, Cambodia, Viet Nam, Taiwan
16.	*A. marshallensis* Stone and Bohart, 1944	Caroline Islands, Marshall Islands, Gilbert Islands
17.	*A. paullusi* Stone and Farner, 1945	Philippines, Malaysia, Indonesia
18.	*A. pernotatus* Farner and Bohart, 1944	New Hebrides
19.	*A. polynesiensis* Marks, 1951	Fiii, Horne Islands, ? Wallis Islands, Ellice Islands, Tokelau Islands, Samoa, Cook Islands, Society Islands, Austral Islands, Marquesas Islands, Tuamotu Archipelago, Pitcairn Island
20.	*A. pseudoscutellaris* (Theobald, 1910)	Fiji
21.	*A. quasiscutellaris* Farner and Bohart, 1944	Solomon Islands
22.	*A. riversi* Bohart and Ingram, 1946	Ryukyu Islands
23.	*A. rotumae* Belkin, 1962	Rotuma Islands
24.	*A. scutellaris* (Walker, 1858)	Indonesia, New Guinea
25.	*A. scutoscriptus* Bohart and Ingram, 1946	Caroline Islands
26.	*A. tabu* Ramalingam and Belkin, 1965	Tonga Islands
27.	*A. tongae* Edwards, 1926	Tonga Islands
28.	*A. upolensis* Marks, 1957	Samoa
29.	*A. varuae* Belkin, 1962	Solomon Islands, Santa Cruz Islands
30.	*Aedes* sp. Wallis form of Belkin, 1962	Wallis Islands
31.	*Aedes* sp. Vanua Lava form of Belkin, 1962	Banks Islands
32.	*Aedes* sp. Tafahi form of Hitchcock and Rozeboom, 1973	Tonga Islands

mind that experiments of different workers, and even those of the same worker at different times, are not always in full agreement. This is partly because of strain differences among species and partly because of different laboratory conditions. Experience in Liverpool has shown that some interspecific crosses are sometimes relatively successful, at other times wholly unsuccessful. The reasons are not yet clear.

Table 2 summarises the compatibility relationships of those species which have been tested. There are two measurements to be taken into account in any cross: the insemination rate and the egg-hatching rate. Information is usually not available on both, and the table gives only an approximation of the relationships based on egg-hatching rates of inseminated females. From the data available, insemination rates of 20-60% are common, and it is noteworthy that *individual* egg batches from inseminated females either show a high hatching rate or all the eggs fail to hatch. In this important respect the hatching pattern differs from that of many *C. pipiens* crosses, in which no fully fertile egg-rafts are produced but in which small proportions of eggs of individual rafts may hatch.

A. polynesiensis x *A. polynesiensis*

Tesfa-Yohannes (1973) examined the relationships of three strains of *A. polynesiensis* from Samoa, Taiaro and Tahiti. Taiaro and Tahiti strains could be crossed easily in both directions giving normal insemination rates and egg-hatching rates. On the other hand, although the Samoan females inseminated by either of the other two strains laid average numbers of eggs, only 5% hatched. The resultant F_1 adults were fully compatible with all parental strains. Eggs from Tahiti females inseminated by Samoan males had a slightly reduced hatching rate.

A. polynesiensis x *A. pseudoscutellaris*

A. polynesiensis and *A. pseudoscutellaris* are closely related species difficult to separate morphologically. Both Woodhill (1954) and Rozeboom and Gilford (1954) showed that successful crosses could be made in both directions, although the egg-hatching rate was only between 5-37%. We have had similar results in Liverpool. The F_1 progeny are fertile and F_2 and F_3 progeny are readily obtainable.

A. polynesiensis x *A. malayensis*

Tesfa-Yohannes and Rozeboom (1974) found that although 10-15% of *A. polynesiensis* females were inseminated by males of *A. malayensis*, no fertile eggs were laid. In Liverpool we have had almost the same experience but on one occasion a successful cross was made. In this experiment 9 of 11 females were inseminated and a small batch of eggs hatched. The F_1 adults were backcrossed to *A. polynesiensis* males and females, but no progeny were obtained. Only 1 of 14 parental females was inseminated by the hybrid males.

The reciprocal parental cross using *A. malayensis* females and *A. polynesiensis* males is more likely to be successful. Tesfa-Yohannes and Rozeboom (1974) crossed three strains of *A. polynesiensis* with *A. malayensis*, and although the insemination rates were only 5-9% and none of the eggs hatched from two of the crosses, the eggs from the third cross, involving Samoan *A. polynesiensis*, gave a high hatching rate.

The hybrid F_1 males were successfully mated to both parental females, but no viable eggs were obtained. The hybrid F_1 females were also backcrossed to the parents and both crosses gave viable eggs. Successive backcrosses to *A. malayensis*, but not to *A. polynesiensis*, were achieved.

In Liverpool the *A. malayensis* female x *A. polynesiensis* male cross has been successful on several occasions, unsuccessful on others, but the backcrosses of the hybrids to *A. polynesiensis* parents have failed to produce progeny.

A. polynesiensis x *A. cooki*

In Liverpool experiments *A. polynesiensis* males readily inseminated *A. cooki* females, but only a single egg has hatched. In the reciprocal cross, on the other hand, most of the inseminated *A. polynesiensis* females laid fertile egg batches. The progeny of these crosses are being investigated.

A. polynesiensis x *A. tabu*

Reciprocal crosses between *A. polynesiensis* and *A. tabu* have been successful. The progeny are currently under investigation.

A. polynesiensis x "Tafahi" form

Hitchcock and Rozeboom (1973) have studied the Samoan population of *A. polynesiensis* and an autogenous unnamed species of the complex from the island of Tafahi, Tonga. Although *A. polynesiensis* females are readily mated by Tafahi males, no viable eggs were obtained, but the reciprocal cross was very successful and the hybrids were inbred for several generations. The F_1 hybrid males could be backcrossed successfully to Tafahi females, but in the backcross to *A. polynesiensis* females, although the insemination rate was high, less than 1% of the eggs hatched. The backcross to *A. polynesiensis* males gave a high hatching rate.

A. pseudoscutellaris x *A. scutellaris*

Woodhill (1950) made a few reciprocal crosses between *A. pseudoscutellaris* and *A. scutellaris*. He did not record whether insemination took place, but all the eggs failed to hatch.

A. pseudoscutellaris x *A. katherinensis*

Woodhill (1950) also tried to cross *A. pseudoscutellaris* and *A. katherinensis* but the eggs from reciprocal crosses failed to hatch.

A. pseudoscutellaris x *A. malayensis*

In Liverpool *A. malayensis* females were readily mated by *A. pseudoscutellaris* males and an insemination rate of 78% has been achieved. However, very few eggs hatched and only two hybrid females have been obtained. The backcross to *A. pseudoscutellaris* males was not successful. The reciprocal parental cross gave a low insemination rate of *A. pseudoscutellaris* females of 2%. One of two egg batches hatched but the backcrosses of the hybrid males and females to *A. pseudoscutellaris* were unsuccessful.

A. scutellaris x *A. malayensis*

Colless (1962) successfully crossed *A. scutellaris* and *A. malayensis* in both directions and both sets of progeny interbred and produced F_2 progeny. No backcrosses were attempted.

A. scutellaris x *A. katherinensis*

The earliest detailed studies of crossing relationships within the complex are by Woodhill (1949, 1950) and Smith-White and Woodhill (1954) using *A. scutellaris* and *A. katherinensis*. Woodhill was the first to observe that whereas the cross between *A. scutellaris* females and *A. katherinensis* males resulted in normal numbers of viable eggs, all the eggs from the reciprocal cross failed to hatch, although the female *katherinensis* had been inseminated. Of the four possible backcrosses of the hybrids to the parents three gave fertile eggs. The exception was the cross between hybrid males

Table 2

Summary of interspecific crossing relationships, based on egg-hatching rates,
within the *Aedes scutellaris* complex

♀ \ ♂	cooki	hebrideus	katherin-ensis	malay-ensis	pernot-atus	polynes-iensis	pseudoscut-ellaris	scut-ellaris	tabu	'Tafahi'
cooki				+		−			++	
hebrideus					+					
katherinensis							−	−		
malayensis	++					+	+	+++	−	
pernotatus		−								
polynesiensis	+++			+			++	+++	+++	−
pseudo-scutellaris			−	+		++		−		
scutellaris			+++	+++		+++	−			
tabu	+++			−		+++				
'Tafahi' form										

+++ high compatibility
++ medium compatibility
+ low compatibility
− incompatible

and *A. katherinensis* females. Woodhill therefore postulated that there was some factor associated with *A. katherinensis* females which made them sterile unless mated with their own males. Smith-White and Woodhill then made a more extensive series of crosses and backcrosses and showed that even after successive backcrosses of (*A. scutellaris* ♀ x *A. katherinensis* ♂) female hybrids to *A. katherinensis* males the infertility of *A. katherinensis* females when mated with the backcross males was retained. The results were very similar to those reported by Laven (1953) from his crosses between strains of the *Culex pipiens* complex, for which a postulate was made that nuclear-independent cytoplasmic factors were responsible for the unidirectional fertility. This phenomenon of cytoplasmic incompatibility in strains is further discussed below.

A. malayensis x *A. cooki*

In reciprocal crosses made in Liverpool between *A. malayensis* and *A. cooki* 23-56% insemination rates were recorded, and small numbers of inseminated females laid eggs which hatched successfully.

A. malayensis x *A. tabu*

In reciprocal crosses made in Liverpool between *A. malayensis* and *A. tabu* insemination rates of 34-57% were recorded, but none of the eggs laid would hatch.

A. cooki x *A. tabu*

In reciprocal crosses in Liverpool between *A. cooki* and *A. tabu* high insemination rates of 64-88% were recorded. The cross between *A. tabu* females and *A. cooki* males produced large numbers of viable eggs, but the reciprocal cross was less successful and only 8 of 37 egg batches hatched.

A. hebrideus x *A. pernotatus*

A. pernotatus females mated readily with *A. hebrideus* males in the laboratory, but none of the eggs hatched (Perry, 1950). In the reciprocal cross, on the other hand, three of 37 *A. hebrideus* females produced eggs which hatched successfully. The 18 hybrid females which were reared were backcrossed to *A. pernotatus* males and 3 produced viable eggs. Most of the backcross progeny died, but 4 males and one imperfect female emerged.

CYTOPLASMIC INCOMPATIBILITY

Incompatibility among populations of the *Culex pipiens* complex is very well documented. Laven (1957, 1967a), in particular, has made large numbers of inter-strain crosses and demonstrated both bidirectional and unidirectional incompatibility as well as bidirectional fertility between different strains. In a small field experiment in Burma Laven (1967b) also demonstrated that cytoplasmic incompatibility had potential as a means of genetic control. Subsequently it was proposed (Laven and Aslamkhan, 1970) that cytoplasmic incompatibility might be integrated with a male-linked translocation in order to provide strains for genetic control experiments, and such strains, with Paris cytoplasm, Delhi genome and male-linked translocations, have now been constructed (Krishnamurthy, 1974).

Unfortunately, incompatibility between strains is not as absolute as was at first thought. For example, Barr (1970) crossed a Californian population with the Italian Scauri strain of *C. pipiens*. The Scauri ♀ x Californian ♂ cross was fully compatible. In the reciprocal cross, however, although most of the egg-rafts failed to hatch, and could be classed as incompatible, a small proportion of rafts had a normal hatching rate and a larger proportion showed a reduced hatch.

A more recent study in Delhi of crossing relationships (Subbarao *et al.*, 1974) has revealed a polymorphism for mating type in wild populations of the *C. pipiens* group. Although the cytoplasm of the Paris and Delhi strains had been reported to show bidirectional incompatibility, Subbarao and her colleagues have now shown that although the majority of Delhi mosquitoes are incompatible with Paris stock in both directions, there is a minority component of the population with males which are fully compatible and females fully incompatible with Paris.

Ageing of the males has also been shown to have an effect on compatibility. Singh *et al.* (in press) in Delhi have demonstrated that with increasing age Paris males show increasing compatibility with Delhi strain females. When the females of these partially compatible matings were reared and successive backcrosses were made to ageing males of the Paris strain, the level of partial incompatibility increased significantly.

If these findings from Delhi, and those of Barr, have a wider application, the interpretation of other laboratory experiments will be made more difficult.

From his studies of incompatibility Laven concluded that the responsible factors were maternally transmitted through the cytoplasm, hence his term cytoplasmic incompatibility, and that the factors were inherited only from the female line through many generations of backcrossing. His hypothesis fits well the results of Smith-White and Woodhill (1954) from their crosses of *A. scutellaris* and *A. katherinensis*. There have been alternative hypotheses to that of Laven, for example those of Smith-White and Woodhill (1954) and McClelland (1967), but the most recent development has been the hypothesis of Yen and Barr (1971, 1973) that incompatibility is related to the presence in the eggs of *C. pipiens* of large numbers of the rickettsia-like symbiont, *Wolbachia pipientis*. They postulated that males and females of a strain of *C. pipiens* carry the same strain of micro-organism and that individuals of different strains may have different organisms. In incompatible crosses the sperm of strain A, when they enter the eggs of females of strain B, are exposed to a foreign strain of organism and are prevented, or incapable, of forming normal diploid embryos. In such cases no progeny are produced except for an occasional parthenogenetic female. In the reciprocal cross the sperm of strain B may be unaffected by the micro-organisms of strain A and normal offspring would be produced. In some cases, where compatibility is said to be partial, a small number of normal offspring are produced from a cross, and Yen and Barr suggest that such a result may be obtained when the micro-organisms do not inhibit all the sperm of the other strain of mosquito and thus allow some survivors to unite with the female nuclei to form normal embryos.

Yen and Barr demonstrated that the micro-organisms could be eliminated by rearing the mosquito larvae in trays containing the antibiotic tetracycline hydrochloride. Owing to the effects of the drug on reproduction, the generation so treated produced few offspring, but the subsequent untreated generations, in which the micro-organisms were still absent, gave normal egg numbers and hatching rates. Mosquitoes in which the symbiont had been removed were termed aposymbiotic. When comparisons were made with formerly incompatible strains, with their symbionts and after their removal, the results were as follows. Males without symbionts became compatible with all females whether or not they had symbionts; and aposymbiotic females mated with males carrying symbionts, whatever their previous relationships, produced no offspring.

Analogies are often drawn between the *C. pipiens* complex and the *A. scutellaris* complex with regard to incompatibility between populations, but work with the latter group lags behind. However, light microscope studies in Liverpool by Dr. E.B. Beckett have shown that bodies which may be rickettsiae are present in the ovaries of some members of the *A. scutellaris* complex, and electron microscopy studies are now in progress to confirm their identity.

Attempts have been made to eliminate by means of antibiotics those putative rickettsiae. Preliminary efforts with tetracycline hydrochloride at concentrations used successfully by Yen and Barr (1973) with *C. pipiens* (0.025-0.05 mg/ml) were not very promising. A more extensive series of experiments by my colleague, Dr. J.O. Wade, using streptomycin, ampicillin, tetracycline, erythromycin, chloramphenicol and rifampicin, produced no decisive improvement in the interspecific fertility of *A. polynesiensis* and *A. malayensis*, but in a few instances tetracycline seemed to show a beneficial effect.

Much remains to be accomplished before our understanding of incompatibility within the *C. pipiens* and *A. scutellaris* complexes is complete. And until we have such an understanding, proposals for manipulating this phenomenon for vector control programmes must remain tentative.

GENETICS OF SUSCEPTIBILITY TO FILARIAE

THE PARASITES

Five species of filariae have been used experimentally to study susceptibility of mosquitoes to infection, *Wuchereria bancrofti, Brugia malayi, B. pahangi, Dirofilaria immitis* and *D. repens*. By far the most important parasite to man is *W. bancrofti*, but since no host other than man is known, experimental work with this species has been restricted. This is the species which is widespread in the South Pacific, where the primary vectors are members of the *A. scutellaris* complex. By means of the freezing method developed for *B. pahangi* by Obiamiwe and Macdonald (1971), we have in Liverpool been preserving in liquid nitrogen the microfilariae of *W. bancrofti* imported from the tropics, and although the survival rate of the microfilariae following treatment is not as high as we should like, the stored material has been suitable for a number of susceptibility tests on mosquitoes.

B. pahangi is a parasite of a variety of mammals in Malaysia, whereas *B. malayi*, which includes both a periodic and a subperiodic form, is a parasite of man and animals in Southeast Asia. Both can be maintained in the laboratory in cats and dogs, but, of the two, *B. pahangi* is the less difficult. Most experimental work on the genetics of infections has therefore been based on *B. pahangi*, but since there is evidence, given below, that susceptibility of *Aedes* to *Wuchereria* is controlled by the same gene as that for *Brugia* it is hoped that the conclusions based on *B. pahangi* will be applicable to *W. bancrofti*.

D. immitis and *D. repens* are parasites of dogs and the work on these species is correspondingly less relevant to the solution of public health problems. Nevertheless, the experimental work on the susceptibility of mosquitoes to these infections supplements our knowledge of vector genetics.

THE MOSQUITO VECTORS

There are many natural vectors of *W. bancrofti*, of which the most important are in the *C. pipiens* complex (for the periodic form of the parasite) and the *A. scutellaris* complex (for the subperiodic form). The principal vector in the latter group is *A. polynesiensis*; several other members of the group have been reported as vectors of local importance on island groups. Most experimental work on genetic aspects of vector susceptibility, however, has been carried out with a mosquito which is not a vector in nature, *A. aegypti*, but which because of its convenience in the laboratory and its genetic variability provides a valuable model for work with the *A. scutellaris* complex.

Aedes aegypti

A single sex-linked recessive gene, designated f^m, controls the susceptibility of *A. aegypti* to *B. malayi, B. pahangi* and *W. bancrofti* (Macdonald, 1962; Macdonald and Ramachandran, 1965). In tests of 43 geographic strains of *A. aegypti* Rodriguez and Craig (1973) found that f^m was absent from 30 of the strains, and the estimated frequency in the remainder varied from 0.10 to 0.73. Most of the strains from East Africa, but none of those from West Africa, carried f^m. However, since many of the strains tested had been maintained in the laboratory for a number of years and may have originated from only a few wild-caught mosquitoes, the reported frequencies may not reflect accurately the true frequencies in the field. In this context it is notable that the strain which originated from Brazzaville in the Congo showed no evidence of f^m, whereas an earlier investigation in the former province of Leopoldville, Belgian Congo, by Henrard *et al.* (1946) showed that 7 of 25 colony *A. aegypti* (presumably of a local strain) were susceptible to *W. bancrofti*.

The position of f^m on the sex chromosomes has been located at 3.4 ± 1.1 crossover units from the sex locus (Macdonald and Sheppard, 1965), and the gene can be transferred between *A. aegypti* strains. The manipulation of the gene would be much easier if male mosquitoes could be scored for susceptibility. This is now possible with the methods of Terwedow and Rodriguez (1973) and Townson (1974, 1975), who have shown by the inoculation of exsheathed microfilariae that males of a susceptible strain of *A. aegypti* are fully susceptible. Unfortunately, a complication which has not yet been resolved has arisen from the experiments of Townson (1974). He has shown that in an apparently fully refractory strain, as determined by tests on a large series of females, a significant proportion of males are susceptible. Work is still in progress to attempt to explain this apparent anomaly.

Macdonald and Ramachandran (1965) showed that susceptibility of *A. aegypti* to *Dirofilaria* infections was not controlled by f^m. Raghavan *et al.* (1967) showed, however, that susceptibility to *D. immitis* infections is heritable and, more recently, Zielke (1973) and McGreevy *et al.* (1974) reported independently that a sex-linked recessive gene, designated *ft* by the latter workers, controlled susceptibility. The location of the gene on the sex chromosomes has not yet been established.

The mode of action of the genes f^m and *ft* are not understood but a study in India dealing with *A. aegypti* susceptible or refractory to *D. immitis* and *D. repens* (National Institute of Communicable Diseases, 1973) reports that susceptible mosquitoes are characterised by high levels of activity of the enzyme alkaline phosphatase. There were no marked differences in the level of acid phosphatase activity in susceptible and refractory mosquitoes.

Culex pipiens complex

Unfortunately the gene controlling susceptibility to *Brugia* in the *C. pipiens* complex does not control susceptibility to *W. bancrofti*. Whereas all *C.p. fatigans* populations tested are, so far as can be established, very susceptible to urban *W. bancrofti*, several tests have shown them to be either refractory to *B. pahangi* (Ogunba, 1969), or to have low infective rates of 4% (Ewert, 1965) or 8.5-25.4% (Desowitz and Chellappah, 1962). *C.p. molestus*, on the other hand, has shown infective rates of 14-19% (Schacher and Khalil, 1965) and 36.3% (Ogunba, 1969). Dr. B.A. Obiamiwe selected a highly susceptible strain from a *C.p. molestus* x *C.p. fatigans* hybrid and made a series of crosses and backcrosses with this stock and refractory *C.p. fatigans*. In a preliminary note, Obiamiwe and Macdonald (1973) reported that susceptibility to *B. pahangi* in the *C. pipiens* complex was controlled by a sex-linked recessive gene which they designated *sb*.

There have been a few unsuccessful attempts to select from vector populations a strain refractory to *W. bancrofti*. For example, Partono and Oemijati (1970) in Jakarta selected for three generations from phenotypically refractory individuals, but although there was a small and perhaps significant reduction in the proportion of susceptible mosquitoes at each generation, there was no evidence of the presence of a major gene for resistance to infection. Singh and Curtis (1974) in Delhi also tried to select a refractory strain from a vector population, but after five generations of selection they concluded that there was no evidence of a gene for non-susceptibility in the original strain. Thomas and Ramachandran (1970) tackled a reciprocal problem. Their *C.p. fatigans* populations in Malaysia had low susceptibility rates of 7-28% to a Malaysian rural periodic strain of *W. bancrofti*, and they attempted to select highly susceptible lines from two of their stocks. Although they appeared to have some success in increasing the susceptibility rates, the numbers of mosquitoes dissected were relatively low. A statistical analysis of the results suggests that additional tests are required to confirm their conclusions.

The results from the work on the *C. pipiens* complex contrast therefore in two main respects with those reported with *A. aegypti*. First, whereas a major gene controls susceptibility to *B. pahangi*, the same gene seems to have no influence on susceptibility to *W. bancrofti*. Second, members of the complex can be highly susceptible to the widespread urban periodic form of *W. bancrofti* but relatively refractory to the rural periodic strain. Therefore, at least two genes, perhaps three, are concerned with susceptibility to *Brugia* and *Wuchereria* infections.

Aedes scutellaris complex

Progress with the genetics of the *A. scutellaris* complex in relation to filarial infections has been slow. The most promising finding has been that *A. malayensis* is refractory to infection with *B. pahangi*, whereas *A. polynesiensis, A. pseudoscutellaris, A. cooki* and *A. tabu*, all of which are vectors of subperiodic *W. bancrofti*, are highly susceptible. Coupled with this finding has been the demonstration that *A. polynesiensis* and *A. pseudoscutellaris* are also susceptible to urban periodic *W. bancrofti* and that *A. malayensis* is refractory to this strain. We have not yet confirmed that *A. malayensis* is refractory to subperiodic *W. bancrofti*. There is a subperiodic strain of *W. bancrofti* on the Nicobar Islands, where *A. malayensis* occurs, but so far only the *Aedes (Finlaya) niveus* group has been incriminated in its transmission (Kalra, 1974). It is of course desirable that the various mosquitoes be tested against several strains of *W. bancrofti* and it is hoped that in the future this will be possible, but for the time being *B. pahangi* must serve as a laboratory model.

The hybrid females of crosses between *A. polynesiensis* and *A. malayensis* have been tested for susceptibility to *B. pahangi* and shown to be refractory. Susceptibility is therefore a recessive trait. Both male and female hybrids have been backcrossed to the *A. malayensis* parents. The backcross progeny from the parental female were tested and 47 out of 47 were refractory. Only four of the progeny of the backcross to the *A. malayensis* male could be tested and these also were refractory. The much more informative backcrosses are those to the *A. polynesiensis* parents but, unfortunately, these we have not yet achieved, although insemination of an *A. polynesiensis* female by a hybrid male was recorded once, and Tesfa-Yohannes and Rozeboom (1974) obtained backcross progeny from their crosses of hybrid females to parental males. The solution of the genetics of susceptibility in the *A. scutellaris* complex must therefore await successful backcrossing. Several promising lines are being followed using *A. cooki* and *A. malayensis.*

   The same perplexing problem as was experienced with males of a 'refractory' stock of *A. aegypti* has been experienced with *A. malayensis,* and Townson (1975) has reported susceptible male *A. malayensis* following inoculation with exsheathed microfilariae of *B. pahangi.* This problem is currently being investigated.

GENETIC CONTROL OF FILARIASIS VECTORS

There are several recent reviews of the various alternative genetic contro᷒. methods which have been proposed for mosquitoes (see, for example, Davidson, 1974; Pal and LaChance, 1974; Pal and Whitten, 1974). In the case of the *C. pipiens* complex, which has been given most attention, five alternatives which may have an application to the *A. scutellaris* complex can be considered. These alternatives involve three components, either alone or in combination: cytoplasmic incompatibility, chromosomal translocations, and genes responsible for resistance to filarial infection.

CYTOPLASMIC INCOMPATIBILITY

In 1967 successful suppression of a small population of *C.p. fatigans* in a village near Rangoon was achieved by the release of males of a strain incompatible with the native mosquitoes (Laven, 1967b). Less successful trials were made in 1972 in India, recorded briefly by Rao (1974) and Pal (1974), and there is no doubt that by itself cytoplasmic incompatibility is not an economic means of suppressing large vector populations. The chief reason is that only males may be released, and the difficulty and the cost of ensuring 100% efficiency in the sexing of the large numbers of mosquitoes which are required for a release programme make the method impractical. The same problem would arise if cytoplasmic incompatibility were considered by itself for suppression of any member of the *A. scutellaris* complex.

CHROMOSOMAL TRANSLOCATIONS

Population suppression by the use of chromosomal translocations, which give a degree of egg sterility in the mosquito progeny, has been postulated by several authors, and Laven (1969) has described the production of translocations in *C. pipiens* and the promising results of some of his cage experiments. There are many advantages in using male-linked translocations, and, with his co-workers, Laven has described the steps leading to a village experiment in Montpellier which was designed to test the effects of introducing such a translocation into a *C. pipiens* population (Laven and Jost 1971; Laven *et al.* 1971; Laven *et al.* 1971a,b). The translocated males were released for two months in 1970 and the frequency of the translocation was monitored during 1971-73 (Cousserans and Guille, 1972, 1974), during which period it declined from 80% in April to less than 1% in September 1973. The results did not fit the earlier predictions of Laven *et al.* (1971a,b) who had expected the frequency to increase. However, Curtis (1975) has since shown that their reasoning had been faulty and that the observed decline agreed with the theoretical expectation.

There was no evidence that the *C. pipiens* population in Montpellier was suppressed. The reduced egg-raft collections in 1971, as compared with 1970, can be explained by a change in the accessibility to the mosquitoes of the primary larval habitat. Furthermore, the egg sterility which was achieved may well have been counterbalanced by higher survival of the larvae owing to density dependent regulation.

Comparable studies to those on *C. pipiens* have been made with *A. aegypti*, and Rai and McDonald (1971), for example, have described the production by irradiation of sex-linked and autosomal translocations and the synthesis and genetics of double translocation heterozygous males. In a small field experiment near Delhi, Rai *et al.* (1973) released male-linked translocation heterozygotes into an *A. aegypti* population and gave evidence that the translocation was successfully introduced into and maintained by the field population. Their experiment was not designed to suppress the population. Some of the advantages of using double translocation heterozygotes for population suppression have been given by Uppal *et al.* (1974) but no field trials have yet been reported with this system.

No attempts have yet been made to induce translocations in the *A. scutellaris* complex but the relative ease with which they can be produced by irradiation in *C. pipiens* and *A. aegypti* suggests that the work should present no great difficulty.

CYTOPLASMIC INCOMPATIBILITY + TRANSLOCATIONS

Laven and Aslamkhan (1970) proposed the integration within *C. pipiens* of cytoplasmic incompatibility and a translocation. It can readily be shown that such an integrated strain would have theoretical advantages. Laven and Aslamkhan concluded that the release of a strain having bidirectional incompatibility with a target population and having, as a result of the translocation, a reproductive potential of only 15% of the normal would lead to eradication of the target population in 3 or 4 generations when the release ratio was only 1:1. The released strain would replace the original population and, it was reasoned, the population size would only reach 15% of the original. Such reasoning is undoubtedly too simplistic since it takes no account of density dependent regulation in the larval populations, nor of the natural selection which would favour individuals with lower rates of sterility than 85%. Laboratory observations have shown that individuals of translocated strains may vary significantly in their sterility and that in unselected stocks the sterility rate may decline (Krishnamurthy, 1974).

An integrated strain of *C.p. fatigans* with Delhi genome and Paris cytoplasm which is bidirectionally incompatible with Delhi mosquitoes (but see p. 10) and which carries a male-linked translocation has been constructed by Krishnamurthy and Laven (in press). This strain, designated IS-31B, was used in trials in three villages in the Delhi area (Rao, 1974) and egg-raft sterility of 50-68% was recorded. A detailed account of this experiment has not yet been seen.

In the future it may be desirable to investigate the possibility of constructing such an integrated strain within the *A. scutellaris* complex. Since there is no incompatibility between strains of *A. aegypti* no comparable work on integrated strains is possible.

TRANSLOCATIONS + GENES FOR RESISTANCE TO FILARIAL INFECTION

Curtis (1968) has theorized on the merits of linking genes for resistance to infections with translocations. The proposal would then be to replace a normal vector population with translocation homozygotes carrying a selected gene. If the translocation could be introduced at a frequency higher than the equilibrium frequency, which would be a function of the relative fertility of the introduced strain and the wild-type, replacement would proceed to fixation for the translocation and the selected gene. Unfortunately, since genes for resistance to infection with *W. bancrofti* have not yet been identified in the *C. pipiens* complex and since no work is being done at present on translocations within the *A. scutellaris* group, this system is unlikely to be evaluated in the near future.

CYTOPLASMIC INCOMPATIBILITY + GENES FOR RESISTANCE TO FILARIAL INFECTION

Bidirectional cytoplasmic incompatibility might serve as a means of replacing a vector population with a population refractory to filarial infection. The principle is the same as for replacement with a cytoplasmic incompatible strain which carries a translocation but whereas the translocation strain would be partially sterile. the non-translocated strain would be fully fertile. Curtis and Adak (1974) have described cage experiments with non-overlapping generations and different release ratios in which they demonstrated the replacement of one or other of two mating types of the *C. pipiens* complex according to the relative frequencies of the two types at the start of the experiments. Although for convenience they used for replacement an incompatible strain with a translocation, they cancelled the effect of the partial sterility by starting each new generation with the same number of larvae from partially sterile rafts as from normal rafts. In this way the translocation was used as a neutral marker which could be considered equivalent to a gene for resistance to infection.

The main advantage of population replacement by means of cytoplasmic incompatibility is that after the new population is established natural selection will operate against wild-type immigrants, provided their number is not too large (see, for example, Laven 1967b). Furthermore, whereas proposals for population suppression have to take account not only of immigrants but of density dependent regulation of larvae, replacement with a fully fertile strain, whose genome will be very largely the same as that of the strain being replaced, does not present this problem. In a number of respects this system looks promising for the *A. scutellaris* complex: incompatibility between species has been established; there is a good chance that a single gene may be responsible for susceptibility to filariae; and the isolated island populations provide ideal targets for genetic control trials. At the present time it would be premature to draw analogies with *C. pipiens* and *A. aegypti* too far, and confirmation of the nature of incompatibility and of monofactorial inheritance of susceptibility are most urgent, but the results and experience derived from both these difficult species encourage the belief that the problems posed by the *A. scutellaris* complex can be overcome.

CONCLUSION

The genetics of the *A. scutellaris* complex promise to be even more interesting and rewarding than those of *C. pipiens* or *A. aegypti*, and the prospects for genetic control of some of the island populations are promising. It is nevertheless too early to present an unduly optimistic picture of these prospects. Apart from the great deal that remains to be done on interspecific incompatibility and on the genetics of filarial susceptibility, account must be taken of the ecology of the vector populations; and, owing to the relative inaccessibility of many of the islands where filariasis is endemic, relatively few ecological studies have been made. If the laboratory experiments during the next year or two confirm the possibility of producing a mosquito with a vector genome minus susceptibility genes within a selected cytoplasm which is incompatible with a vector population, more extensive and intensive field studies will be warranted.

ACKNOWLEDGEMENTS

I am most grateful to Dr. E.B. Beckett, Dr. H. Townson and Dr. J.O. Wade for allowing me to refer to some of their unpublished work and for valuable discussions. I am also indebted to Mr. N.L. Kalra for his confirmation of the identity of *A. malayensis* in the Andaman and Nicobar Islands. The studies in Liverpool have received generous financial support from the World Health Organization and the Wellcome Trust.

REFERENCES.

BARR, A.J. (1970). Partial compatibility and its effect on eradication by the incompatible male method. *Proceedings and Papers of the Thirty-Seventh Annual Conference of the California Mosquito Control Association, Inc. 1969*, pp. 19-24

BELKIN, J.N. (1962). *The mosquitoes of the South Pacific (Diptera, Culicidae)*. Berkeley and Los Angeles: University of California Press

COLLESS, D.H. (1962). Notes on the taxonomy of the *Aëdes scutellaris* group, and new records of *A. paullusi* and *A. albopictus* (Diptera, Culicidae). *Proceedings of the Linnean Society of New South Wales* 87: 312-315

COUSSERANS, J. and GUILLE, G. (1972). Expérience de lutte génétique contre *Culex pipiens* dans la région de Montpellier. 2e année d'observations. *Bulletin biologique de la France et de la Belgique* 106: 337-343

COUSSERANS, J. and GUILLE, G. (1974). Expérience de lutte génétique contre *Culex pipiens* dans la région de Montpellier. Synthèse de quatre années d'observations. *Bulletin biologique de la France et de la Belgique* 108: 253-257

CURTIS, C.F. (1968). Possible use of translocations to fix desirable genes in insect pest populations. *Nature, London* 218: 368-369

CURTIS, C.F. (1975). The behaviour of male-linked translocations in populations. Unpublished document WHO/VBC/75.513

CURTIS, C.F. and ADAK, T. (1974). Population replacement in *Culex fatigans* by means of cytoplasmic incompatibility. I. Laboratory experiments with non-overlapping generations. *Bulletin of the World Health Organization* 51, 249-255

DAVIDSON, G. (1974). *Genetic control of insect pests*. London and New York: Academic Press

DESOWITZ, R.S. and CHELLAPAH, W.T. (1962). The transmission of *Brugia* sp. through *Culex pipiens fatigans*: the effect of age and prior non-infective blood meals on the infection rate. *Transactions of the Royal Society of Tropical Medicine and Hygiene* 56: 121-125

EWERT, A. (1965). Comparative migration of microfilariae and development of *Brugia pahangi* in various mosquitoes. *American Journal of Tropical Medicine and Hygiene* 14: 254-259

HENRARD, C., PEEL, E. and WANSON, M. (1946). Quelques localisations de *Wuchereria bancrofti* Cobbold au Congo Belge. Cycle de développement chez *Culex fatigans* Wied, *Anopheles funestus* Giles, *Aedes aegypti* Linnaeus et *Anopheles gambiae* Giles. *Recueil de Travaux de Sciences Médicales au Congo Belge* **5**: 212-232

HITCHCOCK, J.C. and ROZEBOOM, L.E. (1973). Cross-breeding of *Aedes (S.) polynesiensis* Marks with an autogenous species of the *A. scutellaris* group. *Bulletin of the World Health Organization* **49**: 367-370

HUANG, Y.M. (1972). Contributions to the mosquito fauna of Southeast Asia. XIV. The subgenus *Stegomyia* of *Aedes* in Southeast Asia. I. The *scutellaris* group of species. *Contributions of the American Entomological Institute* **9**: 1-109

KALRA, N.L. (1974). Filariasis among aborigines of Andaman and Nicobar Islands. I. Detection of non-periodic bancroftian filariasis among Nicobarese of Nancowry group of Nicobar Islands. *Journal of Communicable Diseases* **6**: 40-56

KRISHNAMURTHY, B.S. (1974). Construction of "integrated" strains of *Culex pipiens fatigans* Wied. for genetic control. *Journal of Communicable Diseases* **6**: 76-79

KRISHNAMURTHY, B.S. and Laven, H. (In press). Development of cytoplasmically incompatible and integrated (translocated incompatible) strains of *Culex pipiens fatigans* for use in genetic control. *Indian Journal of Medical Research*

LAVEN, H. (1953). Reziprok unterschiedliche Kreuzbarkeit von Stechmücken (Culicidae) und ihre Deutung als plasmatische Vererbung. *Zeitschrift für induktive Abstammungs- und Vererbungslehre* **85**: 118-136

LAVEN, H. (1957). Vererbung durch Kerngene und das Problem der ausserkaryotischen Vererbung bei *Culex pipiens*. II. Ausserkaryotische Vererbung. *Zeitschrift für induktive Abstammungs- und Vererbungslehre* **88**: 478-516

LAVEN, H. (1967a). Speciation and evolution in *Culex pipiens*. In *Genetics of insect vectors of disease*. J.W. Wright and R. Pal (eds.) pp. 251-275. London: Elsevier

LAVEN, H. (1967b). Eradication of *Culex pipiens fatigans* through cytoplasmic incompatibility. *Nature, London* **216**: 383-384

LAVEN, H. (1969). Eradicating mosquitoes using translocations. *Nature, London* **221**: 958-959

LAVEN, H. and ASLAMKHAN, M. (1970). Control of *Culex pipiens pipiens* and *C.p. fatigans* with integrated genetical systems. *Pakistan Journal of Science* **22**: 303-312

LAVEN, H. and JOST, E. (1971). Inherited semisterility for control of harmful insects. I. Productions of semisterility due to translocation in the mosquito, *Culex pipiens* L., by X-rays. *Experientia* **27**: 471-473

LAVEN, H., COUSSERANS, J. and GUILLE, G. (1971a). Expérience de lutte génétique contre *Culex pipiens* dans la région de Montpellier. *Bulletin biologique de la France et de la Belgique* **105**: 357-367

LAVEN, H., COUSSERANS, J. and GUILLE, G. (1971b). Inherited semisterility for control of harmful insects. III. A first field experiment. *Experientia* **27**: 1355-1357

LAVEN, H., MEYER, E., BIENIOK, R., GUILLE, G. and OHMANN, J. (1971). Inherited semisterility for control of harmful insects. II. Degree of sterility and types of translocations in the mosquito *Culex pipiens* L. *Experientia* **27**: 968-969

McCLELLAND, G.A.H. (1967). Speciation and evolution in *Aedes*. In *Genetics of insect vectors of disease*. J.W. Wright and R. Pal (eds.) pp. 277-311. London: Elsevier

MACDONALD, W.W. (1962). The genetic basis of susceptibility to infection with semi-periodic *Brugia malayi* in *Aëdes aegypti*. *Annals of Tropical Medicine and Parasitology* **56**: 373-382

MACDONALD, W.W. and RAMACHANDRAN, C.P. (1965). The influence of the gene f^m (filarial susceptibility, *Brugia malayi*) on the susceptibility of *Aedes aegypti* to seven strains of *Brugia, Wuchereria* and *Dirofilaria*. *Annals of Tropical Medicine and Parasitology* **59**: 64-73

MACDONALD, W.W. and SHEPPARD, P.M. (1965). Cross-over values in the sex chromosomes of the mosquito *Aedes aegypti* and evidence of the presence of inversions. *Annals of Tropical Medicine and Parasitology* **59**: 74-87

McGREEVY, P.B., McCLELLAND, G.A.H. and LAVOIPIERRE, M.M.J. (1974). Inheritance of susceptibility to *Dirofilaria immitis* infection in *Aedes aegypti*. *Annals of Tropical Medicine and Parasitology* **68**: 97-109

MARKS, E.N. (1954). A review of the *Aedes scutellaris* subgroup with a study of variation in *Aedes pseudoscutellaris* (Theobald). *Bulletin of the British Museum (Natural History), Entomology* **3**: 349-414

NATIONAL INSTITUTE OF COMMUNICABLE DISEASES (1973). Studies on histo-chemical basis of differential susceptibility of mosquitoes to parasitic infections. *Annual Report of the National Institute of Communicable Diseases, 1971* pp. 64-68

OBIAMIWE, B.A. and MACDONALD, W.W. (1971). The preservation of *Brugia pahangi* microfilariae at sub-zero temperatures and their subsequent development to the adult stage. *Annals of Tropical Medicine and Parasitology* **65**: 547-554

OBIAMIWE, B.A. and MACDONALD, W.W. (1973). Evidence of a sex-linked recessive gene, *sb*, controlling susceptibility of *C. pipiens* to *B. pahangi*. *Transactions of the Royal Society of Tropical Medicine and Hygiene* **67**: 32-33

OGUNBA, E.O. (1969). The laboratory infection of *Culex pipiens* complex with *Brugia pahangi. Journal of Medical Entomology* **6**: 331-333

PAL, R. (1974). WHO/ICMR programme of genetic control of mosquitos in India. In *The use of genetics in insect control.* R. Pal and M.J. Whitten (eds.) pp. 73-95. London: Elsevier

PAL, R. and LaCHANCE, L.E. (1974). The operational feasibility of genetic methods for control of insects of medical and veterinary importance. *Annual Review of Entomology* **19**: 269-291

PAL, R. and WHITTEN, M.J. (eds.) (1974). *The use of genetics in insect control.* London: Elsevier

PARTONO, F. and OEMIJATI, SRI (1970). Susceptibility of *Culex pipiens fatigans* to *Wuchereria bancrofti* in Djakarta, Indonesia. *Southeast Asian Journal of Tropical Medicine and Public Health* **1**: 515-517

PERRY, W.J. (1950). Biological and crossbreeding studies on *Aedes hebrideus* and *Aedes pernotatus. Annals of the Entomological Society of America* **43**: 123-136

RAGHAVAN, N.G.S., DAS, M., MAMMEN, M.L., SINGH, N.N. and WATTAL, B.L. (1967). Genetic basis of differential susceptibility of *Aedes aegypti* to dirofilarial infection. Part I: Preliminary observations on selection of *Aedes aegypti* strains susceptible and refractory to *Dirofilaria immitis* infection. *Bulletin of the Indian Society for Malaria and other Communicable Diseases* **4**: 318-323

RAI, K.S. and McDONALD, P.T. (1971). Chromosomal translocations and genetic control of *Aedes aegypti*. In *Sterility principle for insect control or eradication.* pp. 437-452. Vienna: International Atomic Energy Agency

RAI, K.S., GROVER, K.K. and SUGUNA, S.G. (1973). Genetic manipulation of *Aedes aegypti*: incorporation and maintenance of a genetic marker and a chromosomal translocation in natural populations. *Bulletin of the World Health Organization* **48**: 49-56

RAO, T.R. (1974). Research on genetic control of mosquitoes in India: review of the work of the WHO/ICMR research unit, New Delhi. *Journal of Communicable Diseases* **6**: 57-72

RODRIGUEZ, P.H. and CRAIG, G.B. Jr. (1973). Susceptibility to *Brugia pahangi* in geographic strains of *Aedes aegypti*. *American Journal of Tropical Medicine and Hygiene* **22**: 53-61

ROZEBOOM, L.E. and GILFORD, B.N. (1954). The genetic relationships of *Aedes pseudoscutellaris* Theobald and *A. polynesiensis* Marks (Diptera: Culicidae). *American Journal of Hygiene* **60**: 117-134

SCHACHER, J.F. and KHALIL, G.M. (1965). *Culex pipiens molestus* as a laboratory vector of *Brugia pahangi*. *Journal of Parasitology* **51**: 806

SINGH, K.R.P. and CURTIS, C.F. (1974). Attempt to select a strain of *Culex pipiens fatigans* Wied. non-susceptible to infection with periodic *Wuchereria bancrofti*. *Journal of Communicable Diseases* **6**: 88-90

SINGH, K.R.P., CURTIS, C.F. and KRISHNAMURTHY, B.S. (In press). Partial loss of cytoplasmic incompatibility with age in males of *Culex fatigans*. *Annals of Tropical Medicine and Parasitology*

SMITH-WHITE, S. and WOODHILL, A.R. (1954). The nature and significance of non-reciprocal fertility in *Aedes scutellaris* and other mosquitoes. *Proceedings of the Linnean Society of New South Wales* **79**: 163-176

SUBBARAO, S.K., CURTIS, C.F., SINGH, K.R.P. and KRISHNAMURTHY, B.S. (1974). Variation in cytoplasmic crossing type in populations of *Culex pipiens fatigans* Wied. from the Delhi area. *Journal of Communicable Diseases* **6**: 80-82

TERWEDOW, H.A. and RODRIGUEZ, P.H. (1973). Development of *Brugia pahangi* in male mosquitoes. *Journal of Parasitology* **59**: 222-223

TESFA-YOHANNES, T.-M. (1973). Genetic relationships of three strains of *Aedes (S.) polynesiensis* Marks. *Journal of Medical Entomology* **10**: 490-492

TESFA-YOHANNES, T.-M. and ROZEBOOM, L.E. (1974). Experimental crossing of *Aedes (S.) polynesiensis* Marks and *A. scutellaris malayensis* Colless (Diptera: Culicidae). *Journal of Medical Entomology* **11**: 323-331

THOMAS, V. and RAMACHANDRAN, C.P.(1970). Selection of *Culex pipiens fatigans* for vector ability to the rural strain of *Wuchereria bancrofti* — a preliminary report. *Medical Journal of Malaya* **24**: 196-199

TOWNSON, H. (1974). The development of *Brugia pahangi* in male *Aedes aegypti* of ' refractory ' genotype. *Annals of Tropical Medicine and Parasitology* **68**: 239-240

TOWNSON, H. (1975). A device for inoculating mosquitoes with larval filariae. *Transactions of the Royal Society of Tropical Medicine and Hygiene* **69**: 12-13

UPPAL, D.K., CURTIS, C.F. and RAI, K.S. (1974). A double translocation heterozygote in *Aedes aegypti*. *Journal of Communicable Diseases* **6**: 98-101

WOODHILL, A.R. (1949). A note on experimental crossing of *Aëdes (Stegomyia) scutellaris scutellaris* Walker and *Aëdes (Stegomyia) scutellaris katherinensis* Woodhill (Diptera, Culicidae). *Proceedings of the Linnean Society of New South Wales* **74**: 224-226

WOODHILL, A.R. (1950). Further notes on experimental crossing within the *Aëdes scutellaris* group of species (Diptera, Culicidae). *Proceedings of the Linnean Society of New South Wales* **75**: 251-253

WOODHILL, A.R. (1954). Experimental crossing of *Aëdes (Stegomyia) pseudoscutellaris* Theobald and *Aëdes (Stegomyia) polynesiensis* Marks (Diptera, Culicidae). *Proceedings of the Linnean Society of New South Wales* **79**: 19-20

YEN, J.H. and BARR, A.R. (1971). New hypothesis of the cause of cytoplasmic incompatibility in *Culex pipiens* L. *Nature, London* **232**: 657-658

YEN, J.H. and BARR, A.R. (1973). The etiological agent of cytoplasmic incompatibility in *Culex pipiens*. *Journal of Invertebrate Pathology* **22**: 242-250

ZIELKE, E. (1973). Untersuchungen zur Vererbung der Empfänglichkeit gegenüber der Hundefilarie *Dirofilaria immitis* bei *Culex pipiens fatigans* und *Aedes aegypti*. *Zeitschrift für Tropenmedizin und Parasitologie* **24**: 34-44

GENETIC FACTORS IN MALARIA PARASITES AND THEIR EFFECT ON HOST-PARASITE RELATIONSHIPS

D. WALLIKER

Institute of Animal Genetics, West Mains Road,
Edinburgh EH9 3JN

INTRODUCTION

The need for a genetic analysis of malaria parasites has been apparent for many years. The emergence of drug-resistance among the human malaria species has underlined the importance of an understanding of parasite factors involved in the evasion of drug action, and of the ways in which these factors are spread in the parasite population. The development of antimalarial vaccines would be greatly facilitated by an understanding of the genetic control of parasite antigens. Until recently, however, genetic studies on malaria parasites have been rarely attempted because the procedures used routinely by geneticists in studying free-living Protozoa have not been easily applicable to parasitic forms.

In order to carry out a genetic analysis of an organism, it is essential that the techniques of making controlled matings between strains can be carried out. In addition, it is important that strains of the organism should be available which exhibit stable differential characteristics, which can be used as genetic markers in crosses. As it is not yet possible to maintain all the stages of the *Plasmodium* life-cycle in *in vitro* culture, the choice of a suitable species for genetic analysis depends on the ease with which it can be kept in laboratory animals. Large numbers of animals are required for establishing clones and for analysing the progeny of crosses particularly when, for example, tests for drug-resistance are to be carried out. For these reasons, the species of *Plasmodium* infecting man and primates cannot yet be employed for such work. Strains of the avian species *Plasmodium gallinaceum* have been used in attempts to demonstrate genetic recombination, but in recent years the species infecting rodents have proved to be the most suitable. A large number of wild isolates of these species are now available (Carter, 1973; Killick-Kendrick, 1974) which can be conveniently maintained in laboratory rodents and cyclically transmitted through mosquitoes.

In this paper an account is given first of some of the techniques which have been.developed for studying genetics of rodent malaria parasites, with a brief description of some of the markers which have been used. Some earlier

25

experiments designed to demonstrate genetic recombination are then discussed, followed by an account of more recent work involving genetic factors in the parasites which influence host-parasite relationships.

GENETIC TECHNIQUES

1. HYBRIDIZATION AND CLONING

The ideal method of hybridizing strains of malaria parasites would be to arrange fertilisation of macrogametes of one strain by microgametes of a second strain. Cloned parasite lines derived from individual parasites at various points in the life-cycle should then be established and examined for recombination of the parent-line characters. However, techniques for separating microgametes from macrogametes are not yet available and satisfactory cloning is possible only when blood forms are used. Although some success in infecting animals with sporozoites from single oocysts has been reported, using mosquitoes infected with only one oocyst (Trembley *et al.*, 1951) and oocysts dissected from mosquito midguts (Walliker, 1972), efforts to establish infections in sufficient numbers for an informative genetic analysis have not so far been successful. Cloning of sporozoites appears to have been attempted only rarely. In the author's laboratory, attempts have been made to infect mice with single sporozoites of *P. chabaudi*. Of 94 animals injected with inocula containing an estimated average of one sporozoite, only one subsequently developed an infection in the blood (Walliker, unpublished observations).

The method which has been developed in Edinburgh for making a genetic analysis of rodent malaria parasites is illustrated in Fig. 1. Mosquitoes are permitted to feed on an animal which has been injected with equal numbers of gametocytes of two parent lines. This allows gametes of each line to undergo cross-fertilisation in the mosquito; self-fertilisation of gametes of each parent line also occurs. The resulting ookinetes, which thus consist of a mixture of hybrid and parental zygotes, are allowed to develop to maturity as oocysts, and the resulting sporozoites are used to establish infections in rodents. The blood forms which emerge in these rodents—the products of the cross—are then examined for recombinant forms. As controls, the parent lines are transmitted through mosquitoes at the same time as the crossed parasites. An additional control may also be made by establishing infections from mixtures of sporozoites of the two lines (see Fig. 1).

The presence of recombinants among the products of a cross may be detected by direct selection pressure on the uncloned parasites, if suitable characters (e.g. differences in drug-sensitivity) distinguish the parent lines, but cloning is necessary for a complete analysis.

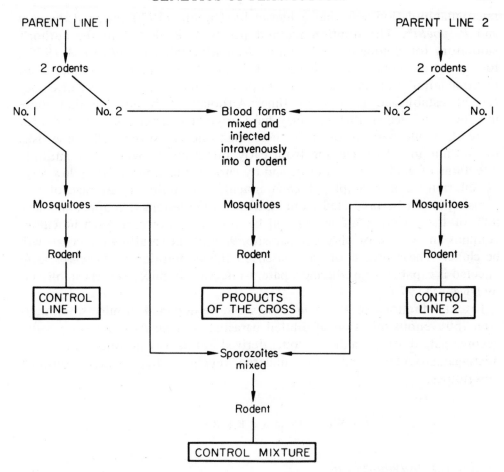

Fig. 1. Procedure used in making cross and in preparation of control samples.

Micro-manipulation and dilution methods have been used for cloning blood forms. Demidowa (1934) obtained infections in two out of 70 birds injected with single parasitised erythrocytes of "*P. praecox*" isolated by micro-manipulation. Coulston and Manwell (1941) used the same technique to clone blood forms of *P. circumflexum*, and succeeded in infecting two out of a total of 18 canaries, although it was not clear whether the isolated erythrocytes contained more than one parasite. Using diluted parasites, five out of ten canaries injected with a calculated average of one parasite became infected. Downs (1947) was able to infect three out of 46 chicks with erythrocytes containing single parasites of *P. gallinaceum* isolated by micro-manipulation, and Bishop (1958) used the same method to establish *P. gallinaceum* clones in thirteen birds out of a total of 46 injected. The first success in cloning erythrocytic forms of rodent malaria parasites by micro-manipulation was that achieved by Diggens (1970) using *P. berghei* and *P. yoelii**. The dilution method has been exploited in the author's laboratory for cloning *P. yoelii* and *P. chabaudi* (Walliker *et al.*, 1973, 1975); for genetic work this method is considered more suitable than micro-manipulation as it is simpler in practice and a large number of clones can be established in a short time. Although it is possible that some infections derived in this way may have originated from cells infected with more than one parasite or from more than one parasitised cell, these risks can be minimised by cloning from early infections in which few multiple infections of erythrocytes occur, and by choosing an appropriately low level of dilution. For example, if each inoculum contains an average of one parasite, it can be predicted from statistical calculations that approximately 58% of the resulting infections will be clones. If, however, each inoculum contains an average of only 0.1 parasite, 96% of the resulting infections will be clones. These predictions are based on the assumption that each parasite injected is capable of producing a patent infection in mice, as was established by Diggens (1970).

Patent infections of *P. yoelii* clones can be detected in mice seven days after intravenous injection of diluted parasites. *P. chabaudi* clones normally become patent after ten days. Clones derived in this way produce macro- and micro-gametocytes, and can undergo cyclical transmission through mosquitoes.

2. GENETIC MARKERS

(a) Enzyme polymorphism

Studies on numerous organisms have shown that the electrophoretic mobility of enzymes is frequently a rich source of stable genetic variation. As enzyme forms identified in this way represent the products of single genetic loci, important genetic information can be obtained from studies of their recombination and segregation in crosses. Among free-living Protozoa, enzyme variation has been used in genetic studies on *Paramecium* (Tait, 1968, 1970a, 1970b) and *Tetrahymena* (Allen and Gibson, 1973).

Using starch gel electrophoresis, Carter (1970) first detected enzyme variation among isolates of *P. berghei* and *P. yoelii*. Later (Carter, 1973; Carter and Walliker, 1975) extensive variation was found among enzymes of other rodent malaria species, notably in *P. chabaudi* isolates. The technique was also used to identify enzyme variation in *P. falciparum* (Carter and

---

* The taxonomic nomenclature of *P. berghei* and *P. yoelii* used in this paper is that proposed by Killick-Kendrick (1974).

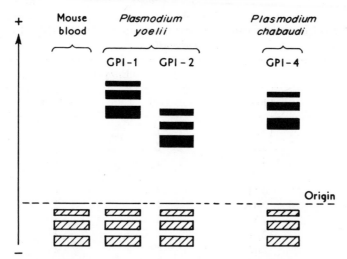

Fig. 2. Electrophoretic forms of glucose phosphate isomerase (GPI) characteristic of *Plasmodium yoelii* and *Plasmodium chabaudi*, using the Tris HCl, pH 8.0 system of starch gel electrophoresis (Carter, 1973). Dark bands represent parasite enzymes, and hatched bands represent host forms.

McGregor, 1973). The most suitable enzymes for analysis by this technique were glucose phosphate isomerase (GPI), 6-phosphogluconate dehydrogenase (6PGD) and lactate dehydrogenase (LDH). The variant forms of GPI found among *P. yoelii* and *P. chabaudi* isolates are illustrated diagrammatically in Fig. 2. Each variant form of each enzyme is allocated a number; thus, in *P. yoelii* isolates two forms of GPI are found—GPI-1 and GPI-2. Each species of *Plasmodium* was found to possess its own characteristic enzyme forms. Table 1 lists the forms of GPI, 6PGD and LDH found among isolates of *P. yoelii* and *P. chabaudi*.

(b) Drug-resistance

Resistance to most of the commonly used anti-malarial drugs has now been recorded among the human malaria species (for reviews see Peters, 1970, 1974). The stability of the resistance varies according to the drug used and the presence or absence of drug pressure. Resistance to 4-aminoquinolines such as chloroquine has frequently proved to be unstable in the absence of drug pressure, while resistance to antifolates such as proguanil and pyrimethamine and to sulphonamides such as sulphadiazine is usually stable. Resistance to drugs of the latter two groups is therefore the most suitable for use in genetic work.

   Resistance to antifolates has been developed in many species of

Table 1

Distribution of electrophoretic forms of enzymes among selected lines of *P. yoelii* and *P. chabaudi*

Species	Line	Enzymes		
		GPI	6PGD	LDH
P.y. yoelii	17X	1	1	1
	33X	2	1	1
P.y. killicki	194ZZ	1	1	1
P.y. nigeriensis	N67	2	1	1
P. chabaudi	6AL	4	2	2
	3AR	4	2	3
	47AS	4	2	3
	32CR1	4	2	3
	2BJ	4	2	4
	57AF	4	2	5
	10AJ	4	3	2
	8BC	4	3	4
	10BK	4	3	4
	3CQ	4	3	5

Plasmodium by numerous workers. Notable examples of the stability of this type of resistance are given by Bishop and McConnachie (1950), who passaged a proguanil-resistant line of *P. gallinaceum* 140 times through untreated chicks with no apparent loss in resistance, and Greenberg and Bond (1954) who developed a pyrimethamine-resistant line of *P. gallinaceum* which maintained its resistance for at least six months in the absence of drug pressure. Among the rodent species, Diggens (1970), Walliker *et al.* (1973) and Morgan (1974) produced pyrimethamine-resistant lines of *P. berghei* and *P. yoelii* which were stable after many blood and mosquito transfers. In each of these three studies, resistant lines were produced in a single step, by exposure of sensitive parasites to a single course of treatment with the drug at a high dose. The production of resistant lines by this method from cloned sensitive parasites (Bishop, 1962; Morgan, 1974), the low frequency with which these lines appear and their stability in passage suggest strongly that resistance to antifolates arises by mutation rather than by adaptation.

Parasite lines resistant to pyrimethamine have been exploited in genetic recombination experiments involving other markers using lines of *P. gallinaceum* and of rodent malaria species. This work will be discussed later in this paper.

(c) Other markers

Other characters differentiating parasite strains which have been used in genetic work include differences in the development of exoerythrocytic forms of strains of *P. gallinaceum* (Greenberg and Trembley, 1954a, 1954b; Trembley and Greenberg, 1954), host-specificity (Yoeli *et al.*, 1969), strain-specific cross-immunity (Oxbrow, 1973) and virulence of blood forms (Yoeli *et al.*, 1975). Each of these investigations will be discussed in more detail in the following sections.

GENETIC RECOMBINATION EXPERIMENTS

To obtain evidence that hybridization of parasite lines has occurred during a cross, it is necessary to identify the presence of non-parental parasite types among the progeny. In addition, it is important to carry out a series of control experiments to ensure that the new phenotype has arisen by hybridization and not by a genetic change in one of the parent lines, such as mutation. Experimental attempts to demonstrate genetic recombination have been made using *P. gallinaceum* and rodent malaria species.

1. P. GALLINACEUM

Greenberg and Trembley were the first to attempt to detect genetic recombination in malaria parasites derived from mosquitoes which had fed on a mixture of two strains. In a series of experiments they made use of strains derived from a common parent *P. gallinaceum* strain, which had become differentiated from one another in their mode of development during prolonged laboratory passage. In their first experiments (Greenberg and Trembley, 1954a; Trembley and Greenberg, 1954) no evidence of hybridization was found, as no non-parental forms developed. In their next experiment (Greenberg and Trembley, 1954b), mixed infections of a pyrimethamine-resistant Bl strain and a sensitive M strain were passaged through mosquitoes. The BI strain, when transmitted through mosquitoes by itself, produced only exoerythrocytic forms in the recipient chicks. The M strain produced normal erythrocytic forms after mosquito passage. After transmission of the mixed infection, erythrocytic forms were recovered which were resistant to pyrimethamine, suggesting that cross-fertilisation between the BI and M strains had occurred. Alternative explanations were that the M strain had become drug-resistant by mutation, or that the BI strain had changed its pattern of development.

The chief disadvantage of using these strains in genetic work was that they were derived from a common parent strain. The growth characteristics of these strains were frequently unstable. This variability was discussed by Garnham (1966) who pointed out that "when *P. gallinaceum* is induced to live in a variety of unnatural conditions, it seems to lose its capacity to produce gametocytes, to produce no malaria pigment in erythrocytic schizonts, to develop in haemopoietic cells and to grow exclusively with or without phanerozoites. Probably few of these substrains represent true mutations, because after a number of normal transmissions most of them will regain the character of the type". These considerations apply also to the subsequent work reported by Greenberg (1956) on mixed infections of the BI and SP strains of *P. gallinaceum.*

2. RODENT MALARIA PARASITES

(a) Cross-fertilisation of gametes

The first demonstration of genetic recombination in rodent malaria parasites following cross-fertilisation of gametes was made in 1971 (Walliker *et al.,* 1971), using two lines of *P. yoelii.* A mixed infection of line A, which was pyrimethamine-resistant and possessed enzyme-form GPI-1, and line C which was drug-sensitive and possessed enzyme-form GPI-2, was passaged through mosquitoes. Drug-treatment of the products of the cross revealed the presence of GPI-2 as well as GPI-1 in the surviving parasites (Table 2).

Table 2

Enzyme analysis following pyrimethamine treatment of products of the cross between lines A and C of *P.y. yoelii,* and control infections

	GPI-type	
	Untreated parasites	Treated parasites
Products of the cross	1 and 2	1 and 2
Control line A	1	1
Control line C	2	—
Control sporozoite mixture	1 and 2	1

Control tests on the parent lines alone and on infections derived from sporozoite mixtures of the two lines showed that the drug-resistant GPI-2 parasites had been produced by cross-fertilisation and not by mutation of the parent line C or any other gene transfer mechanism. In later work (Walliker *et al.,* 1973), the alternative recombinant form (pyrimethamine-sensitive, GPI-1) was detected by cloning the products of crosses. A high proportion of recombinants was found among these clones, indicating that the parent lines had readily undergone cross-fertilisation.

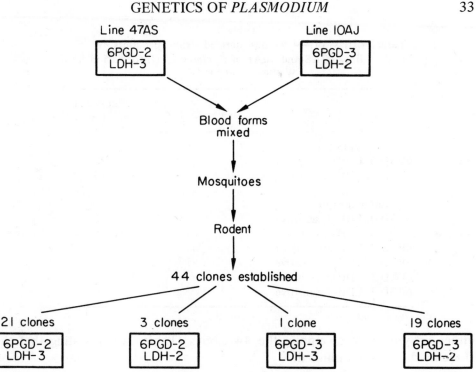

Fig. 3. The inheritance of forms of 6PGD and LDH in a cross between lines 47AS and 10AJ of *P. chabaudi*.

In similar experiments with *P. chabaudi*, crosses were made between two lines differing by two enzyme markers, as well as by pyrimethamine-sensitivity (Walliker *et al.*, 1975). The two parent lines were line 47AS, characterised by 6PGD-2, LDH-3 and pyrimethamine-resistance, and line 10AJ characterised by 6PGD-3, LDH-2 and pyrimethamine-sensitivity. A study of the inheritance of the enzyme-forms was made by cloning the progeny of the cross (Fig. 3). 44 clones were established, each of which showed only one form of each enzyme; in none were two forms of the same enzyme found together. Four clones showed recombination between enzyme-forms, three being characterised by 6PGD-2/LDH-2 and one by 6PGD-3/LDH-3. These results showed, therefore, that recombination and segregation of the parental enzyme forms had occurred before the emergence of parasites into the blood, observations which demonstrated that the blood forms were genetically haploid. This conclusion supports the growing cytological evidence (Sinden and Canning, 1973; Canning and Sinden, 1973) that a reduction division probably occurs during development of the oocyst.

The pyrimethamine-resistance character segregated independently of

D. WALLIKER

Table 3

Characteristics of 44 clones derived from products of cross between lines 47AS and 10AJ of *P. chabaudi* (Information from Walliker *et al.*, 1975)

	Number of clones isolated
Parental types	
6PGD-2, LDH-3, resistant	20
6PGD-3, LDH-2, sensitive	14
Recombinant types	
6PGD-2, LDH-3, sensitive	1
6PGD-3, LDH-2, resistant	5
6PGD-2, LDH-2, resistant	2
6PGD-2, LDH-2, sensitive	1
6PGD-3, LDH-3, resistant	1
6PGD-3, LDH-3, sensitive	0

either enzyme marker among the 44 clones (Table 3), suggesting that the three markers were unlinked.

(b) Synpholia

An unusual method of non-gametic exchange of genetic material termed "synpholia" was proposed by Yoeli *et al.* (1969) following results obtained from mixed infections of *P. vinckei* and *P. berghei* strains. Blood forms of a pyrimethamine-resistant strain of *P. vinckei* which was not infective to hamsters and a drug-sensitive strain of *P. berghei* infective to hamsters were permitted to develop together in a mouse for five days. Parasites from this animal were then injected into twelve hamsters which were treated with varying doses of pyrimethamine. Pyrimethamine-resistant *P. berghei* was detected in six of the treated hamsters.

The explanation given by Yoeli *et al.* (1969) for this result was that during the mixed infection of the two species in the donor mouse, transfer of pyrimethamine-resistance from the *P. vinckei* to the *P. berghei* strain had occurred when trophozoites of each had developed together within the same erythrocyte. The most likely alternative explanation was that a mutation to pyrimethamine-resistance had occurred in the *P. berghei* strain. The mutation rate to pyrimethamine-resistance has been estimated for *P. berghei* as 1.75×10^{-11} (Schoenfeld *et al.*, 1974) and for *P. yoelii* as 2.3×10^{-11} (Morgan, 1974). Mutation rates of this order could not account satisfactorily for the appearance of resistant mutants in six of the twelve hamsters used by

Yoeli *et al.*, unless the mutation event had occurred in the donor mouse. If this were the case, however, it might be expected that the progeny of the mutant would have been distributed to each of the twelve hamsters. No evidence for "synpholia" was found in the work of Walliker *et al.* (1973) and Schoenfeld *et al.* (1974), but in neither of these studies were the exact procedures used by Yoeli *et al.* followed. The true explanation for "synpholia", therefore, remains enigmatic at present.

GENETIC FACTORS INFLUENCING HOST-PARASITE RELATIONSHIPS

1. STRAIN-SPECIFIC IMMUNITY

The genetic control of antigenic variation is a subject of clear importance in host-parasite relationships in malaria as in other protozoan infections. There is ample evidence of extensive antigenic diversity in *P. falciparum* isolates, revealed by immuno-diffusion techniques (Wilson *et al.*, 1969). Antigenic variants detectable by schizont agglutination tests are known to occur during *P. knowlesi* infections (Brown *et al.*, 1968). These variants appear to be produced by antibody-induced phenotypic changes rather than by selection of pre-existing mutants (Brown, 1974), although cloned infections have not yet been studied. Work on species of *Plasmodium* which are amenable to genetic analysis has had to rely on relatively insensitive serological tests such as cross-protection and passive transfer of immune serum. Some of this work has indicated antigenic variation during *P. berghei* infections (Cox, 1959; Briggs and Wellde, 1969), and cross-immunity experiments have successfully distinguished some of the rodent malaria species (Cox and Voller, 1966). Antigenic differences between strains of two subspecies of *P. yoelii* were detected in similar tests by Oxbrow (1973), which formed the basis for the only genetic investigation of strain-specific immunity carried out so far.

The work of Oxbrow involved *P. y. nigeriensis* strain N67 and *P. y. yoelii* strain 17X. Mice immunised with each strain were protected against challenge by the homologous strain. However, while immunization with strain N67 protected against 17X as well as N67, immunization with 17X did not prevent infection by N67; N67 was able to grow in 17X—immunized animals, although to a lower level than in control infections. It appeared, therefore, that strain-specific cross-immunity factors in these parasites controlled their ability to grow in immunized hosts.

The genetic basis of these factors was investigated in a cross between strains N67 and 17X. The two strains differed from one another additionally in enzyme and drug-sensitivity markers. N67 possessed enzyme-forms GPI-2

Table 4

Characteristics of 16 clones derived from cross between *P.y. yoelii* strain N67
(Information from Oxbrow, 1973)

		Survival in mice immunized to strain 17X	Drug response	GPI-type	Number of clones isolated
Parental types	{	No	Resistant	1	3
	{	Yes	Sensitive	2	7
Recombinant types	⎧	No	Sensitive	2	1
	⎪	Yes	Resistant	1	2
	⎨	No	Sensitive	1	3
	⎪	Yes	Resistant	2	0
	⎪	No	Resistant	2	0
	⎩	Yes	Sensitive	1	0

and was sensitive to pyrimethamine, while 17X possessed enzyme-form GPI-1 and was pyrimethamine-resistant. After cross-fertilisation of the two strains in mosquitoes, the products of the cross were cloned. 16 clones were established and examined for each of the parental characters (Table 4). Two of these showed characteristics of strain 17X (GPI-1, resistant) but were able to grow in mice immunized to 17X, and one showed N67 characteristics (GPI-2, sensitive) and was unable to grow in these animals. Three further clones were recombinants involving the enzyme and drug-sensitivity markers (GPI-1, sensitive) and were unable to grow in immunized mice.

These results indicated strongly that factors determining the ability of these strains to grow in immunized mice were able to undergo genetic recombination with the other markers. The precise nature of these factors remains a subject for further investigation; some preliminary work by Oxbrow (1973) suggested that the greater natural virulence of strain N67 could not fully account for its growth in the immunized mice. It is hoped that more precise serological tests for identifying antigenically distinct parasites will soon become available for use with rodent plasmodia, in order that this important subject can be investigated further.

2. VIRULENCE

Variations in the virulence of strains of *Plasmodium* are well-known to most malariologists. Strains which normally undergo a mild course of infection may become virulent during routine passage and, similarly, virulent infections may sometimes revert to mildness (Alger *et al.*, 1971). Some of the factors known to cause alterations in the normal course of parasitaemia of malaria parasites are as follows:-

(a) *Mistaken identity of strain.* The risks involved when more than one strain of parasite is being passaged in laboratory animals need no emphasis here. A pertinent comment by Walker (1966) is that "the identity of morphologically indistinguishable strains of trypanosomes and malaria depends more on the label on the mouse box than on the strain itself".

(b) *Prolonged blood passage.* An increase in virulence frequently results from continuous blood passage (e.g. Yoeli *et al.*, 1966). Occasionally, strains become less virulent during prolonged passage (e.g. Carrescia and Arcolea, 1957).

(c) *Host diet.* Dietary deficiency of the host may result in a less severe infection. An essential growth requirement for the parasite, but not its host, is p-aminobenzoic acid (PABA). Jacobs (1964) demonstrated the effect of different dietary concentrations of PABA on *P. berghei* infections in mice.

(d) *Host age.* Mice become less susceptible to *P. yoelii* infections with advancing age (Oxbrow, 1969). This observation can probably be explained by the relatively fewer numbers of reticulocytes in older mice, which are preferentially invaded by this species.

(e) *Concurrent infections.* A concurrent infection with another organism may alter the normal course of parasitaemia of malaria parasites. Well-known examples are the effects on rodent parasites of infections by *Ererythrozoon coccoides* and *Haemobartonella muris* (Peters, 1965; Ott *et al.*, 1967) and by oncogenic viruses (Salaman *et al.*, 1969).

(f) *Genetic factors in the host.* In man, a number of genes affecting red cells, such as the autosomal gene for haemoglobin S and the sex-linked gene for glucose-6-phosphate dehydrogenase deficiency, are known to be involved in resistance to malaria (Luzzatto, 1974); immune response genes have also been the subject of recent study (Ceppellini, 1973). In rodent malaria, the strain of mouse used is known to influence the course of infection (Greenberg *et al.*, 1954; Most *et al.*, 1966) although the genetic basis of these differences is not understood.

(g) *Genetic factors in the parasite.* When each of the above factors has been taken into account, there remain examples of variations in virulence which are probably the result of genetic differences between parasite strains. An example of genetically determined virulence was reported by Yoeli *et al.* (1975), when the normally mild strain 17X of *P. y. yoelii* underwent a sudden enhancement in virulence following the removal of a stabilate from the deep-freeze. An investigation into the nature of this virulence and its effect on the host has now been undertaken (Walliker *et al.*, 1976) and some of the first results are discussed below.

The blood forms of *P. y. yoelii* strains normally invade reticulocytes in preference to mature red cells. Parasitaemias build up slowly, to reach a peak of around 50% by the fifteenth day of infection, after which a rapid decrease occurs, parasites becoming sub-patent after three weeks (Fig. 4). The virulent line differs from the parent strain 17X in its capacity for development in mature erythrocytes. Parasites invade reticulocytes by preference for the first two days of infection, but then enter mature erythrocytes, a parasitaemia of 90% being attained by the fifth day (Fig. 4). Infected animals normally die by the seventh day. The virulence of the line is maintained after blood and mosquito passages, a feature which suggests that

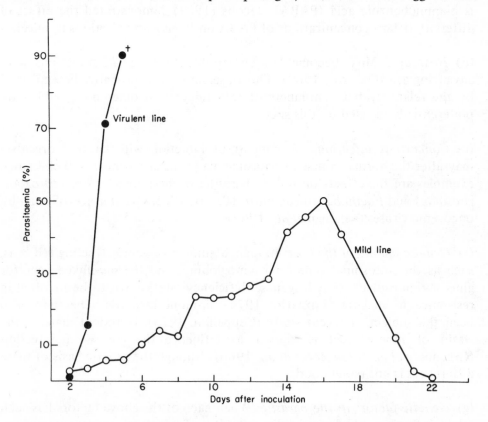

Fig. 4. The course of infection of virulent and mild lines of *P. y. yoelii* in C57 Black mice. † represents death of host.

Table 5

Characteristics of 56 clones derived from cross between virulent
and mild lines of *P.y. yoelii*.

	Number of clones isolated
Parental types	
GPI-1, sensitive, virulent	15
GPI-2, resistant, mild	5
Recombinant types	
GPI-1, sensitive, mild	1
GPI-2, resistant, virulent	10
GPI-1, resistant, mild	5
GPI-2, sensitive, virulent	3
GPI-1, resistant, virulent	9
GPI-2, sensitive, mild	5
Clones showing atypical development	
GPI-1, resistant (Clone 54)	1
GPI-1, sensitive (Clone 55)	1
GPI-2, resistant (Clone 56)	1

a genetic change in the parasite was responsible for its altered characteristics.

A study of the enzyme-patterns of the virulent line revealed forms typical of a number of strains of *P. y. yoelii* including strain 17X, a finding which showed that no mistake in strain identity had taken place. Host strain and age, and dietary factors were excluded from being the primary causes of the virulence as the differences in infection patterns between virulent and mild lines were maintained in inbred mice of similar age given a standardised PABA diet. Concurrent infections with other organisms were also excluded from being the primary cause, as no acquisition of virulence by a mild line took place during its development in a mixed infection with the virulent line.

In genetic experiments, crosses were made between the virulent line and a mild line, and studies made on the recombination and segregation of the virulence character with other markers. The other markers were enzyme and drug-sensitivity differences, the virulent line being GPI-1 and pyrimetha-mine-sensitive, and the mild line GPI-2 and drug-resistant. After cross-fertilisation in mosquitoes, 56 clones were established from the progeny, which were examined for each of the parent-line markers (Table 5). The virulent character appeared to be inherited in simple Mendelian fashion, having recombined with each of the other markers. All possible recombinant forms were represented among the clones, suggesting possibly that the three characters were unlinked.

In addition to clones which exhibited clearly defined mild or virulent patterns of infection, there were three which developed in an atypical manner. In one (clone 54), extensive invasion of mature erythrocytes took place, but no host deaths resulted. In the other two (clones 55 and 56) the virulent character was expressed in some mice but not in others; parasites taken from mice with mild infections continued to develop in a mild form in subsequent passages. The explanation for these cases of atypical virulence remains to be determined. It is possible that further mutations to virulence had occurred in certain mice, although this seems unlikely as no virulent forms were detected in control infections involving the mild line. Another possible explanation is that genetic recombination events during the cross had given rise to parasites exhibiting unstable virulence, similar to that seen in, for example, strain N67 of *P. y. nigeriensis*; blood forms of this strain commonly infect mature erythrocytes in some mice, but not others (Killick-Kendrick, 1973). A third possibility is that host factors were involved which caused a suppression of virulence in certain mice.

The feature which most clearly distinguishes the virulent line from mild *P. y. yoelii* lines is its ability to develop extensively in mature erythrocytes after an initial preference for reticulocytes. Whether this is due to the inability of merozoites of mild lines to penetrate mature erythrocytes or to their inability to develop to maturity within them remains to be determined. Reduction of the PABA concentration in the host's diet causes the virulent line to become mild, parasites remaining restricted to reticulocytes (Walliker, unpublished observations). This demonstrates the interaction of genetic factors in the parasite and environmental factors in the host for the full expression of the virulent character.

A final important feature of infections with the virulent line is that mice which die from the infection show heavy blockage of brain capillaries, similar to that seen in cases of cerebral malaria in man (Yoeli and Hargreaves, 1974). There are a number of hypotheses to explain the physiological processes involved in cerebral malaria (reviewed by Maegraith and Fletcher, 1972), but little is known of the role of parasite factors. The work discussed here demonstrates the importance of a genetic change in the parasite as a cause of virulence; it is hoped that further investigations will reveal how the genetic factors involved contribute to the processes leading to brain capillary blockage.

ACKNOWLEDGEMENTS

Support for much of the work described in this paper was provided by a grant from the Medical Research Council to Professor G.H. Beale. A research grant from the Scientific Council of N.A.T.O. is also gratefully acknowledged.

REFERENCES

ALGER, N.E., BRANTON, M., HARANT, J. and SILVERMAN, P.H. (1971). *Plasmodium berghei* NK65 in the inbred A/J mouse: variations in virulence of *P. berghei* demes. *Journal of Protozoology* **18**: 598-601.

ALLEN, S.L. and GIBSON, I. (1973). Genetics of *Tetrahymena*. In *Biology of Tetrahymena*. A.M. Elliott (ed.), pp. 307-373. Stroudsburg, Pennsylvania: Dowden, Hutchinson and Ross Inc.

BISHOP, A. (1958). An analysis of the development of resistance to metachloridine in clones of *Plasmodium gallinaceum*. *Parasitology* **48**: 210-234.

BISHOP, A. (1962). An analysis of the development of resistance to proguanil and pyrimethamine in *Plasmodium gallinaceum*. *Parasitology* **52**: 495-518.

BISHOP, A. and McCONNACHIE, E.W. (1950). The stability of paludrine resistance in *Plasmodium gallinaceum* in the absence of the drug. *Parasitology* **40**: 159-162.

BRIGGS, N.T. and WELLDE, B.T. (1969). Some characteristics of *Plasmodium berghei* "relapsing" in immunised mice. *Military Medicine* **134**: 1243-1248.

BROWN, K.N. (1974). Antigenic variation and immunity to malaria. In *Parasites in the immunised host: mechanisms of survival*. CIBA Foundation Symposium **25**: 35-51. Amsterdam: Elsevier, Excerpta Medica.

BROWN, I.N., BROWN, K.N. and HILLS, L.A. (1968). Immunity to malaria; the antibody response to antigenic variation by *Plasmodium knowlesi*. *Immunology* **14**: 127-138.

CANNING, E.U. and SINDEN, R.E. (1973). The organization of the ookinete and observations on nuclear division in oocysts of *Plasmodium berghei*. *Parasitology* **67**: 29-40.

CARRESCIA, P.M. and ARCOLEA, G. (1957). Importanza della virulenza del ceppo di *Plasmodium berghei* nel determinare infezion; ad andamento rapido nei topi albini. *Rivista di Malariologia* **36**: 65-72.

CARTER, R. (1970). Enzyme variation in *Plasmodium berghei*. *Transactions of the Royal Society of Tropical Medicine and Hygiene* **64**: 401-406.

CARTER, R. (1973). Enzyme variation in *Plasmodium berghei* and *Plasmodium vinckei*. *Parasitology* **66**: 297-307.

CARTER, R. and McGREGOR, I.A. (1973). Enzyme variation in *Plasmodium falciparum* in the Gambia. *Transactions of the Royal Society of Tropical Medicine and Hygiene* **67**: 830-837.

CARTER, R. and WALLIKER, D. (1975). New observations on the malaria parasites of rodents of the Central African Republic; *Plasmodium vinckei petteri* subsp. nov. and *Plasmodium chabaudi* Landau, 1965. *Annals of Tropical Medicine and Parasitology* **69**: 187-196.

CEPPELLINI, R. (1973). Specific immune response genes and defence against malaria. In *Abstracts of the 9th International Congress on Tropical Medicine and Malaria, Athens 1973*. p. 267.

COULSTON, F. and MANWELL, R.D. (1941). Single parasite infections and exoerythrocytic schizogony in *Plasmodium circumflexum*. *American Journal of Hygiene* **34**: 119-125.

COX, H.W. (1959). A study of relapse *Plasmodium berghei* infection isolated from white mice. *Journal of Immunology* **82**: 209-214.

COX, F.E.G. and VOLLER, A. (1966). Cross-immunity between the malaria parasites of rodents. *Annals of Tropical Medicine and Parasitology* **60**: 297-303.

DEMIDOWA, L.W. (1934). Ueber die geringste zur erzeugung der experimentellen malaria nötige *Plasmodium praecox* Zahl. *Giornale di Batteriologia e Immunologia* **13**: 872-877.

DIGGENS, S.M. (1970). 1. Single-step production of pyrimethamine-resistant *P. berghei.* 2. Cloning erythrocytic stages of *P. berghei. Transactions of the Royal Society of Tropical Medicine and Hygiene* **64**: 9-10.

DOWNS, W.G. (1947). Infections of chicks with single parasites of *Plasmodium gallinaceum* Brumpt. *American Journal of Hygiene* **46**: 41-44.

GARNHAM, P.C.C. (1966). *Malaria parasites and other Haemosporidia.* Oxford: Blackwell Scientific Publications.

GREENBERG, J. (1956). Mixed lethal strains of *Plasmodium gallinaceum*: drug-sensitive, transferable (SP) x drug-resistant, non-transferable (BI). *Experimental Parasitology* **5**: 359-370.

GREENBERG, J. and BOND, H.W. (1954). Resistance of a pyrimethamine-resistant strain of *Plasmodium gallinaceum* to certain 2,4 diamino-pyrimidines and related compounds. *Journal of Parasitology* **40**: 472-475.

GREENBERG, J. and TREMBLEY, H.L. (1954a). Infections produced by mixed strains of *Plasmodium gallinaceum* in chicks. *Journal of Parasitology* **40**: 336-340.

GREENBERG, J. and TREMBLEY, H.L. (1954b). The apparent transfer of pyrimethamine-resistance from the BI strain of *Plasmodium gallinaceum* to the M strain. *Journal of Parasitology* **40**: 667-672.

GREENBERG, J., NADEL, E.M. and COATNEY, G.R. (1954). Differences in survival of of several inbred strains of mice and their hybrids infected with *Plasmodium berghei. Journal of Infectious Diseases* **95**: 114-118.

JACOBS, R.L. (1964). Rôle of p-amino benzoic acid in *Plasmodium berghei.* infection in the mouse. *Experimental Parasitology* **15**: 213-225.

KILLICK-KENDRICK, R. (1973). Parasitic protozoa of the blood of rodents. 1. The life-cycle and zoogeography of *Plasmodium berghei nigeriensis* subsp. nov. *Annals of Tropical Medicine and Parasitology* **67**: 261-277.

KILLICK-KENDRICK, R. (1974). Parasitic protozoa of the blood of rodents: a revision of *Plasmodium berghei. Parasitology* **69**: 225-237.

LUZZATTO, L. (1974). Genetic factors in malaria. *Bulletin of the World Health Organization,* **50**: 195-202.

MAEGRAITH, B. and FLETCHER, A. (1972). The pathogenesis of mammalian malaria. *Advances in Parasitology* **10**: 49-75.

MORGAN, S. (1974). *The genetics of malaria parasites: studies on pyrimethamine-resistance.* Ph.D. Thesis, University of Edinburgh.

MOST, H.M., NUSSENZWEIG, R.S., VANDERBERG, J., HERMAN, R. and YOELI, M. (1966). Susceptibility of genetically standardised (JAX) mouse strains to sporozoite- and blood-induced *Plasmodium berghei* infections. *Military Medicine* **131**: (Supplement) 915-918.

OTT, K.J., ASTIN, J.K. and STAUBER, L.A. (1967). *Eperythrozoon coccoides* and rodent malaria: *Plasmodium chabaudi* and *Plasmodium berghei. Experimental Parasitology* **21**: 68-77.

OXBROW, A.I. (1969). Some growth characteristics of *Plasmodium berghei* strains. *Transactions of the Royal Society of Tropical Medicine and Hygiene* **63**: 6.

OXBROW, A.I. (1973). Strain-specific immunity to *Plasmodium berghei*: a new genetic marker. *Parasitology* **67**: 17-27.

PETERS, W. (1965). Competitive relationship between *Eperythrozoon coccoides* and *Plasmodium berghei* in the mouse. *Experimental Parasitology* **16**: 158-166.

PETERS, W. (1970). *Chemotherapy and drug-resistance in malaria.* London and New York, Academic Press.

PETERS, W. (1974). Recent advances in antimalarial chemotherapy and drug-resistance. *Advances in Parasitology* **12**: 69-114.

SALAMAN, M.H., WEDDERBURN, N. and BRUCE-CHWATT, L.J. (1969). The immunodepressive effect of a murine plasmodium and its interaction with murine oncogenic viruses. *Journal of General Microbiology* **59**: 383-391.

SINDEN, R.E. and CANNING, E.U. (1973). Ultra-structure and cytochemistry of nuclear division in *Plasmodium. Progress in Protozoology* p. 385. (Abstracts of papers read at the Fourth International Congress of Protozoology. Clermont-Fernand, 1973).

SCHOENFELD, C., MOST, H. and ENTNER, N. (1974). Clermont-Ferrand, 1973). malaria: transfer of resistance vs. mutation. *Experimental Parasitology* **36**: 265-277.

TAIT, A. (1968). Genetic control of β-hydroxybutyrate dehydrogenase in *Paramecium aurelia. Nature, London* **219**: 941.

TAIT, A. (1970 a). Genetics of NADP-dependent isocitrate dehydrogenase in *Paramecium aurelia. Nature, London* **225**: 181-182.

TAIT, A. (1970b). Enzyme variation between syngens in *Paramecium aurelia. Biochemical Genetics* **4**: 461-470.

TREMBLEY, H.L. and GREENBERG, J. (1954). Further studies on the hybridisation of strains of *Plasmodium gallinaceum. Journal of Parasitology* **40**: 475-479.

TREMBLEY, H.L. GREENBERG, J. and COATNEY, G.R. (1951). Strain differences in *Plasmodium gallinaceum* Brumpt. II. Experiences with the sporozoite and single oocyst passage of the BI strain. *Journal of the National Malaria Society* **10**: 68-75.

WALKER, P.J. (1966). Freeze preservation of parasitic protozoa. *Laboratory Practice* **15**: 423-426.

WALLIKER, D. (1972). An infection of *Plasmodium berghei* derived from sporozoites of a single oocyst. *Transaction of the Royal Society of Tropical Medicine and Hygiene* **4**: 543.

WALLIKER, D., CARTER, R. and MORGAN, S. (1971). Genetic recombination in malaria parasites. *Nature, London* **232**: 561-562.

WALLIKER, D., CARTER, R. and MORGAN, S. (1973). Genetic recombination in *Plasmodium berghei. Parasitology* **66**: 309-320.

WALLIKER, D., CARTER, R. and SANDERSON, A. (1975). Genetic studies on *Plasmodium chabaudi*: recombination between enzyme markers. *Parasitology* **70**: 19-24.

WALLIKER, D., SANDERSON, A., YOELI, M. and HARGREAVES, B.J. (1976). A genetic investigation of virulence in a rodent malaria parasite. *Parasitology* (In press).

WILSON, R.J.M., McGREGOR, I.M., HALL, P., WILLIAMS, K. and BARTHOLOMEW, R. (1969). Antigens associated with *Plasmodium falciparum* infections in man. *The Lancet* **2**: 201-205.

YOELI, M., NUSSENZWEIG, R., UPMANIS, R.S. and MOST, H. (1966). Resistance of *Plasmodium chabaudi* infected mice to a fulminating and fatal strain of *Plasmodium vinckei. Nature, London* **211**: 49-51.

YOELI, M., UPMANIS, R.S. and MOST, H. (1969). Drug-resistance transfer among rodent plasmodia. 1. Acquisition of resistance to pyrimethamine by a drug-sensitive strain of *Plasmodium berghei* in the course of its concomitant development with a pyrimethamine-resistant *P. vinckei* strain. *Parasitology* **59**: 429-447.

YOELI, M. and HARGREAVES, B.J. (1974). Brain capillary blockage produced by a virulent strain of rodent malaria. *Science* **184**: 572-573.

YOELI, M., HARGREAVES, B., CARTER, R. and WALLIKER, D. (1975). Sudden increase in virulence in a strain of *Plasmodium berghei yoelii*. *Annals of Tropical Medicine and Parasitology* **69**: 173-178.

GENETICS OF THE HOST-PARASITE RELATIONSHIP BETWEEN *BIOMPHALARIA GLABRATA* AND *SCHISTOSOMA MANSONI*

CHARLES S. RICHARDS

Laboratory of Parasitic Diseases,
National Institute of Allergy and Infectious Diseases,
National Institutes of Health,
Bethesda, Maryland 20014, USA

INTRODUCTION

Investigators studying the host-parasite relationship between *Biomphalaria glabrata* and *Schistosoma mansoni* have reported differences in susceptibility to infection between various geographic stocks and hybrids of *B. glabrata* and differences in infectivity between various geographic strains and hybrids of *S. mansoni* (Files and Cram, 1949; Kuntz, 1952, with an Egyptian strain of *S. mansoni*; Barbosa and Barreto, 1960, with several Brazilian stocks of *B. glabrata*; Paraense and Correa, 1963). Most of these studies have dealt with adults only and with populations rather than with individuals with infection frequencies ranging from 0% to 100%. However, Newton in 1953 demonstrated susceptibility in juvenile snails of a Brazilian stock of *B. glabrata*, the adults of which were refractory to a Puerto Rican strain of *S. mansoni.*

Results of studies such as these suggest that most natural populations of *B. glabrata* and *S. mansoni* are heterogenic, consisting of individuals varying in either susceptibility or infectivity. Differences in various snail and parasite populations could be the result of qualitative differences in genetic alleles and quantitative differences in gene frequencies. In our experiment we have isolated snails and allowed them to reproduce by self-fertilization. Juveniles and adults were then selected through successive generations of clonal stocks until consistent susceptibility characteristics were obtained. Controlled crosses were subsequently made between snails of different susceptibility types to analyze the genetic factors involved.

In the case of the parasite *S. mansoni*, individual miracidia have been tested for infectivity and selection made through successive generations in an attempt to derive strains showing consistent differences in infectivity.

Characteristics making *B. glabrata* well suited for genetic studies were reviewed by Richards (1973a). *B. glabrata* is hermaphrodite and isolated snails reproduce by self-fertilization. However, when two snails are mated, reciprocal cross-fertilization temporarily suppresses self-fertilization. Pigmentation, with three alleles, serves as a genetic marker for controlled crosses: wild type black pigmentation is dominant, albino recessive, and "blackeye" recessive to wild type but dominant over albino. It is possible to self an albino and then mate it to four or more different snails in series, alternating wild type and blackeye mates. A wild type or blackeye snail can be used as a male in matings with several (15-20) albino snails in series. Such serial matings yield results very helpful in analyzing the genetics of invisible characters such as susceptibility to infection.

Snail stocks, parasite strains, and methods involved have been described by Richards (1973b, 1975a, 1975b) and by Richards and Merritt (1972, 1975). Testing and selection, using both juvenile and adult snails and two strains of *S. mansoni* (PR=Puerto Rican; L=St. Lucian) resulted in seven susceptibility types (Fig. 1). Crosses suggested that juvenile susceptibility to the PR strain is determined by a complex of several genetic factors (Richards and Merritt, 1972). All susceptible snail stocks are not genetically alike, and

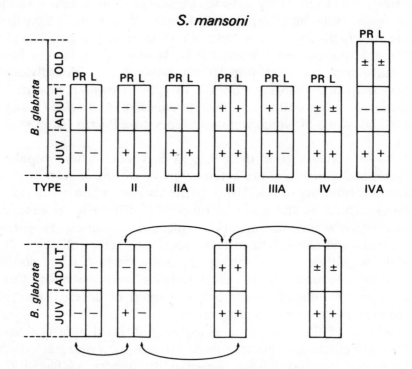

Fig. 1. Genetic variations in susceptibility to infection of *B. glabrata*, with age and with exposure, to two different strains of *S. mansoni*, Puerto Rican (PR) and St. Lucian (L). Susceptibility differences which have been studied by controlled crossing experiments are indicated in the lower part of the figure. Unsusceptible = −, Susceptible = +.

they may carry unexpressed genes for insusceptibility; similarly, refractory stocks may carry unexpressed genes for susceptibility. Adult susceptibility, in snails whose juveniles are susceptible to PR *S. mansoni*, is determined by a single genetic factor with insusceptibility dominant. In some snail stocks additional genetic factors modify adult susceptibility causing variable results.

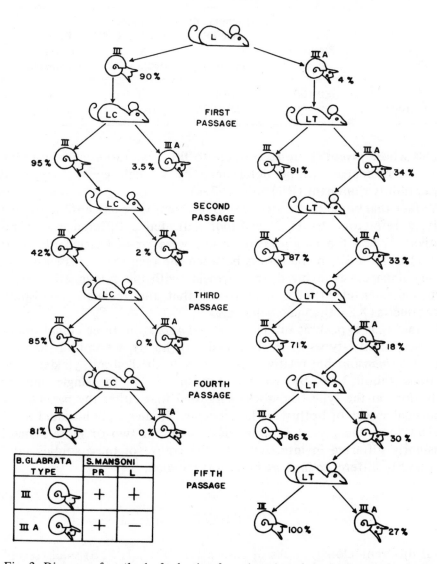

Fig. 2. Diagram of method of selection for substrains of the St. Lucian (L) strain of *S. mansoni*. Type III "control" *B. glabrata*, susceptible to the parent L strain are depicted as albinos; type IIIa "test" snails, essentially refractory to the parent L strain are depicted as blackeye *B. glabrata*. Percentage infections in snails exposed individually to single miracidia is shown.

Table 1
Results of reciprocal crosses between Puerto Rican and St. Lucian *S. mansoni.*

B. glabrata susceptibility types	Percentage infection frequencies in juvenile snails exposed to one miracidium per snail with observed penetration			
		F$_1$ miracidia from crosses		
	Parent PR strain *S. mansoni*	male PR X female L	female PR X male L	Parent L strain *S. mansoni*
IIIa	80-100	19	1.7	4
III (controls)	80-100	80-100	80-100	80-100

In snails whose juveniles are susceptible to PR *S. mansoni*, susceptibility to the L strain appears to be determined by a single genetic factor with insusceptibility dominant (Richards, 1975a).

The fact that some clonal stocks of *B. glabrata* were susceptible to PR but relatively refractory to L *S. mansoni* indicated a difference in parasite infectivity. When the two parasite strains were crossed (Richards, 1975b: Table 1) differences in the results between the reciprocal crosses suggested that sex linkage was involved, thus agreeing with the cytogenetic results of Short and Menzel (1960), who found that the female schistosome is heterogametic (XY), the male being XX.

The fact that exposures of juvenile *B. glabrata* from three clonal stocks of two susceptibility types (Fig. 1; 2 and 3a), highly susceptible to the PR strain of *S. mansoni* but relatively refractory to the L strain, yielded a few L infections (about 7% by routine exposures, 4% by single miracidial penetrations in the type IIIa stock) suggested that either the parasite strain or the snail stocks or both were heterogenic. Studies were initiated in order to select from the parent L strain of *S. mansoni* two or more substrains consistently differing in infectivity. In the course of these studies another susceptibility difference in *B. glabrata* was revealed.

METHODS

Several different clonal stocks of susceptible (Figs. 1, 2, 3) snails served as controls to demonstrate potential infectivity of miracidia. The type IIIa stock provided "test" snails refractory to most L strain miracidia. Snails of each type were exposed to single miracidia of the parent L *S. mansoni* strain. Cercariae from paired, infected "control" snails were injected into mice.

Table 2

Selection for a substrain (Lc) less infective than the parent L strain of *S. mansoni.*

Cercariae injected from type III snails female X male	Mouse Number	Snail infections (1 miracidium per snail)	
		Type IIIa "test" snails infected/exposed	Type III "control" snails infected/exposed
1st passage			
Lc-11 X Lc-5	28	5/32	6/7
Lc-15 X Lc-5	31*	0/29	12/12
Lc-6 X Lc-14	23*	0/75	5/5
Lc-6 X Lc-14	38	0/15	4/5
Lc-6 X Lc-10	35*	0/46	11/11
		5/197 (3.5%)	38/40 (95%)
2nd passage			
Lc-31-4 X Lc-31-5	21	1/27	4/14
Lc-31-4 X Lc-23-1	19	1/28	9/17
Lc-23-2 X Lc-23-1	0-2	0/9	
Lc-23-2 X Lc-31-5	0-5	0/7	
Lc-23-2 X Lc-35-4	15	0/27	8/15
Lc-31-7 X Lc-35-4	3-5	0/33	
Lc-31-9 X Lc-35-4	3-7	2/38	
Lc-35-11 X Lc-35-6	5-4*	0/41	13/25
		4/210 (2%)	34/71 (42%)
3rd passage			
Lc-5-4-6 X Lc-5-4-1	12-4	0/20	1/3
Lc-5-4-3 X Lc-5-4-1	12-2	0/20	6/7
Lc-5-4-5 X Lc-5-4-9	15-3	0/40	12/13
Lc-5-4-3 X Lc-5-4-7	14-3*	0/40	10/11
		0/120 (0%)	29/34 (85%)
4th passage			
Lc-14-3-7 X Lc-14-3-6	27-1	0/20**	10/10
Lc-14-3-10 X Lc-14-3-1	25-6	0/28	37/48
		0/48 (0%)	47/58 (81%)

* source of parasites for next passage
** snails exposed to 5 miracidia per snail

Control and test snails were exposed to single miracidia from the resulting crosses in the mice, with observed penetration. Cercariae from paired surviving control snails infected by those miracidia from individual mice which gave the lowest frequencies of infection in test snails, were injected into mice. This selection, for a "control" Lc substrain of *S. mansoni* consistently less infective than the parent L strain, is in the fourth such

Table 3

Selection for a substrain (Lt) more infective than the parent L strain of *S. mansoni*.

Cercariae injected from type IIIa snails female X male	Mouse Number	Snail infections (1 miracidium per snail)	
		Type IIIa "test" snails infected/exposed	Type III "control" snails infected/exposed
1st passage			
Lt-3 X Lt-5	3*	24/54	12/13
Lt-7 X Lt-5	7*	6/24	7/8
Lt-7 X Lt-6	8	8/35	9/10
		38/113 (34%)	28/31 (91%)
2nd passage			
Lt-3-2 X Lt-3-3	0-8	9/30	13/15
Lt-7-3 X Lt-3-3	0-25*	13/37	13/15
		22/67 (33%)	26/30 (87%)
3rd passage			
Lt-0-25-4 X Lt-0-8-1	8-8*	3/25	
Lt-0-25-4 X Lt-0-25-7	8-5	9/39	24/30
Lt-0-25-4 X Lt-0-25-3	7-3*	6/40	11/19
Lt-0-25-2 X Lt-0-25-3	7-2	4/17	
		22/121 (18%)	35/49 (71%)
4th passage			
Lt-8-8-1 X Lt-8-8-3	17-5*	15/40	16/20
	17-5*	55/84** (66%)**	
Lt-7-3-1 X Lt-8-8-3	18-2	9/39	40/45
		24/79 (30%)	56/65 (86%)
5th passage			
Lt-17-5-2 X Lt-17-5-3	29-1	8/30 (27%)	30/30 (100%)

* source of parasites for next passage
** snails exposed to 5 miracidia per snail

passage (Fig. 2 and Table 2). Cercariae from paired, infected, type IIIa test snails were also injected into mice. Control and test snails were exposed to single miracidia from the resulting crosses in the mice and penetration was observed. Cercariae from paired, infected, test snails were again injected into mice. This selection for a "test" Lt substrain of *S. mansoni* more infective than the parent L strain is in the fifth such passage (Fig. 2 and Table 3). In some experiments, groups of type IIIa test snails were also exposed to 5 miracidia for comparison with those exposed to single miracidia.

It has been our experience that, in the absence of continual testing and selection, snail stocks genetically refractory to *S. mansoni* have generally been more stable than susceptible stocks. In studies on infectivity in *S. mansoni*, seven different type III susceptible stocks of *B. glabrata* were used as control snails as a precaution. Three of these which showed increasingly inconsistent results were eliminated. One of the remaining stocks (now designated IIIb) differs consistently from the other three, being insusceptible to one of the derived substrains of the parent L strain of *S. mansoni*, suggesting another genetic susceptibility difference.

RESULTS

SELECTION FOR A "CONTROL" SUBSTRAIN LESS INFECTIVE THAN THE PARENT L STRAIN OF *S. MANSONI*

Following the first series of injections in mice of cercariae from susceptible type III control snails, miracidia from five crosses were tested (Table 2, Fig. 2). Single miracidial penetrations infected 0%-16% (mean 3.5%) of the test snails and 95% of the control snails. With the second passage in mice, miracidial penetrations infected 0%-6% (mean 2%) of the test snails but only 42% of the controls. After the third passage in mice, single miracidial penetrations infected 0% of 120 test snails (also none of 123 test snails exposed to 5 miracidia per snail became infected) but infected 85% of the control snails. Infections from miracidia from one mouse (14-3 in Table 2) provided cercariae for injection in to another group of mice as a substrain designated Lc. Following this fourth passage, miracidia were infective to type III control snails but non-infective to type IIIa.

SELECTION FOR A "TEST" SUBSTRAIN MORE INFECTIVE THAN THE PARENT L STRAIN OF *S. MANSONI*

Following the first series of injections in mice of cercariae from Type IIIa test snails, single miracidial penetrations infected 23%-45% (mean 34%) of the test snails but 91% of the controls (Table 3, Fig. 2). After the second passage in mice, single penetrations infected 30%-35% (mean 33%) of the test snails, and 87% of the control snails. Following the third passage single miracidial penetrations infected 12%-24% (mean 18%) of the test snails and 71% of the control snails—and after the fourth passage single miracidial penetrations infected 23%-37.5% (mean 30%) of the test snails and 86% of the control snails. Miracidia from mouse 17-5 infected (mean 37.5%) 15/40 of the test snails by single miracidial penetrations and 66% (55/84) by routine exposures to 5 miracidia per snail. Following the fifth passage, miracidia have so far infected 27% of the test snails and 100% of the control snails.

SNAIL SUSCEPTIBILITY TO L SUBSTRAINS
OF *S. MANSONI*

One of the susceptible control snail stocks (now designated IIIb) was found to be refractory to miracidia from mouse 14-3 of the third passage of the control substrain of L *S. mansoni.* Cercariae from other control snails exposed to miracidia from mouse 14-3 were used for the fourth passage in mice to establish the Lc substrain. Most type IIIb snails tested refractory to miracidia from this fourth passage. Both type IIIa and a selected clonal stock of IIIb snails tested were susceptible to PR *S. mansoni* but refractory to the Lc substrain (Fig. 3). Infection frequencies in type IIIb snails exposed to the Lt substrain were higher (85%) than in type IIIa snails (about 30%).

DISCUSSION

The substrains designated Lc and Lt have been derived from the parent L strain of *S. mansoni.* At the current stage of selection in these substrains, type IIIa "test" snails show 0% infection by single miracidial penetrations with the Lc substrain and about 30% infections with the Lt substrain, as compared to the original 4% infections with the parent L strain (Fig. 3).

The Lc substrain is still infective to type III susceptible snails. One of the snail stocks used as controls, on the basis of previous susceptibility results,

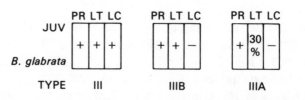

Fig. 3. Results of exposures of individual juvenile (JUV) *B. glabrata* of three susceptibility types to single miracidia of the Puerto Rican and the St. Lucian Lt and Lc substrains of *S. mansoni* with observed penetration; plus marks (+) indicate 80-100% infection frequencies.

was refractory to the Lc substrain but highly susceptible to the Lt substrain, and has been designated type IIIb (Fig. 3).

Infection results of the Lt substrain in test snails suggest that this substrain still includes miracidia of two infectivity types. Following the fourth passage in mice, single miracidial penetrations resulted in infections in 30% of the test snails, while 66% of a group of test snails exposed to 5 miracidia per snail became infected. This suggests that miracidia of the Lt substrain vary in their infectivity.

These studies have involved only a few geographic populations of one host species (*B. glabrata*) and only two geographic strains of one parasite species (*S. mansoni*). However, the results suggest considerable intraspecific genetic variation in host susceptibility and parasite infectivity. Studies on other populations of these species may reveal additional genetic variations, and comparable genetic variations may be anticipated in other host and parasite species. Thus the potential for intraspecific genetic variations must be considered when analyzing results of experimental host-parasite studies; the conclusions expressed or implied by other workers may be incorrect if the possibility of genetic variation was not considered.

ACKNOWLEDGEMENTS

The assistance of Mr. Paul C. Shade and Mr. Thomas A. Hallack, Jr. in these studies is gratefully acknowledged.

REFERENCES

BARBOSA, F.S. and BARRETO, A.C. (1960). Differences in susceptibility of Brazilian strains of *Australorbis glabratus* to *Schistosoma mansoni*. *Experimental Parasitology* **9**: 137-140.

FILES, V.S. and CRAM, E.B. (1949). A study on the comparative susceptibility of snail vectors to strains of *Schistosoma mansoni*. *Journal of Parasitology* **35**: 555-560.

KUNTZ, R.E. (1952). Exposure of planorbid snails from the Western Hemisphere to miracidia of the Egyptian strain of *Schistosoma mansoni*. *Proceedings of the Helminthological Society of Washington* **19**: 9-15.

NEWTON, W.L. (1953). The inheritance of susceptibility to infection with *Schistosoma mansoni* in *Australorbis glabratus*. *Experimental Parasitology* **2**: 242-57.

PARAENSE, W.L. and CORREA, L.R. (1963). Variation in susceptibility of populations of *Australorbis glabratus* to a strain of *Schistosoma mansoni*. *Revista do Instituto de Medicina Tropical de Sao Paulo* **5**: 15-22.

RICHARDS, C.S. (1973a). Genetics of *Biomphalaria glabrata* (Gastropoda: Planorbidae). *Malacological Review* **6**: 199-202.

RICHARDS, C.S. (1973b). Susceptibility of adult *Biomphalaria glabrata* to *Schistosoma mansoni* infection. *American Journal of Tropical Medicine and Hygiene* **22**: 748-56.

RICHARDS, C.S. (1975a). Genetic factors in susceptibility of *Biomphalaria glabrata* for different strains of *Schistosoma mansoni. Parasitology* **70**: 221-241.

RICHARDS, C.S. (1975b). Genetic studies on variation in infectivity of *Schistosoma mansoni. Journal of Parasitology* **61**: 233-36.

RICHARDS, C.S. and MERRITT, J.W. Jr. (1972). Genetic Factors in susceptibility of juvenile *Biomphalaria glabrata* to *Schistosoma mansoni* infection. *American Journal of Tropical Medicine and Hygiene* **21**: 425-34.

RICHARDS, C.S. and MERRITT, J.W. Jr. (1975). Variation in size of *Biomphalaria glabrata* at maturity. *The Veliger* **17**: 393-95.

SHORT, R.B. and MENZEL, M.Y. (1960). Chromosomes of nine species of schistosomes. *Journal of Parasitology* **46**: 273-87.

HYBRIDIZATION OF SCHISTOSOMES AND SOME OF ITS IMPLICATIONS

C.A. WRIGHT and V.R. SOUTHGATE

British Museum (Natural History), Cromwell Road,
London SW7 5BD

INTRODUCTION

As a sequel to a study of *Schistosoma intercalatum* and its systematic affinities (Wright *et al.*, 1972) an experiment was started to investigate the results of hybridization between *S. intercalatum* and the possibly closely related species *S. mattheei.* Some preliminary observations were made concerning the relationships between hybrid larval schistosomes and their snail hosts (Wright, 1974) but at about the same time a focus of natural hybridization between *S. intercalatum* and *S. haematobium* was discovered in Cameroon (Wright *et al.*, 1974; Southgate *et al.*, in press). This discovery led to an intensification of the laboratory experiments to provide data for use in interpretation of the field observations and these data are also providing a background for reappraisal of earlier work on the hybridization of schistosomes.

Schistosomes, being dioecious, lend themselves more readily to breeding experiments than do other digenetic trematodes, all of which are hermaphrodite. The technique for performing such experiments is theoretically very simple in that the sex of the adult worms is genetically determined. Thus, although there is as yet no simple method for detecting the sex of any of the larval stages it is known that all of the cercariae derived from a single miracidium will develop into adults of the same sex. A number of snail hosts for each parasite species are exposed individually to a single miracidium and rodents are subsequently exposed to cercariae emanating from two snails only, each carrying larvae from a different parasite. In practice the logistics of such experiments are complicated by the high failure rate at each stage of the cycle. It is necessary to expose large series of snails in order to ensure that enough become infected, infection rates of 10% are considered quite good when single miracidia are used, also, because the sex of living cercariae cannot be determined, there are inevitably a number of final host infections in which the worms of both species are of the same sex. Given these problems and the fact that a single complete cycle of most of the species takes three to four months there are considerable limitations to progress. Nevertheless, the results which are currently being obtained have both theoretical and practical interest.

55

HISTORICAL

Vogel (1941 and 1942) carried out cross-breeding experiments with the three principal schistosome parasites of man, *S. mansoni*, *S. haematobium* and *S. japonicum*. These studies were concerned more with the factors which affect maturation of the adult worms in the definitive hosts than they were with hybridization In fact Vogel obtained no definite evidence of hybridization from any of the matings which he achieved, but he did find that females of some species which failed to mature in the absence of males would reach maturity and produce eggs of limited viability when paired with males of another species. The progeny from these females showed only maternal characteristics and he attributed them to parthenogenesis, induced by some hormonal or nutritional factor derived from contact with worms of the opposite sex. The hormonal theory had been postulated earlier by Severinghaus (1928) as a result of his work on *S. japonicum*. The stimulus provided by males of other species to maturation and egg-production by *S. mansoni* females was further demonstrated by Short (1948) using males of *Schistosomatium douthitti* and by Armstrong (1965) with *Schistosomatium douthitti* and *Heterobilharzia americana* but in all cases the eggs produced by the *S. mansoni* females were of very low viability. In contrast, Short (1952a and b) found that pairing of *Schistomatium douthitti* had no apparent effect on the rate of maturation of either sex and unpaired females produced viable eggs. These eggs were smaller than those produced by paired females, their infectivity for snails was lower but viable cercariae were produced. The cercariae gave rise to both male and female worms, suggesting that the females of this species are probably heterogametic. Short (1957) confirmed this by demonstrating a hetermorphic pair of chromosomes in *Schistosomatium douthitti* and subsequently Short and Menzel (1959) showed that all female cercarial embryos of this species had both X and Y chromosomes and all male embryos were either haploid X or diploid XX. A triploid XXY proved to be male, suggesting that the female-determining influence of the Y chromosome is not particularly strong. Short and Menzel (1960) later examined the chromosomes of nine other species of schistosomes but only in *Ornithobillharzia canaliculata* were they able to demonstrate a heteromorphic pair of chromosomes in the female. A stage intermediate between the failure to develop of unpaired female *S. mansoni* and the successful parthenogenesis of *Schistosomatium douthitti* has been reported by Taylor *et al.* (1969) for *S. mattheei*. In this species the females reach maturity in single sex infections but they lay very small, non-viable eggs. If paired with male *S. mansoni* they produce eggs of normal shape and size for *S. mattheei* but with reduced viability and no evidence of hybridization.

All of the cross-pairings mentioned so far were performed between species which are not considered to be particularly closely related and some form of apomixis or pseudogamy rather than hybridization appears to have been responsible for egg-production. Le Roux (1954a) described successful experimental cross-mating of *S. mansoni* with the related species *S. rodhaini*, a parasite of rodents in Africa. Here all of the evidence pointed to hybridization. The cross was viable in both directions, the F_1 eggs were intermediate in shape between those of the parental species and the F_1 miracidia were reported to have a wider intermediate host range than those of *S. rodhaini*. Le Roux considered that these results from the two African species with lateral spines on their eggs might suggest the possibility of hybridization between members of the species complex with terminal-spined eggs. Interbreeding between these species could provide an explanation for the occasional finding, in human infections of *S. haematobium*, of eggs similar to those of species normally parasitic in ungulates. In the same year Le Roux (1954b) reported such a case in which eggs of *S. mattheei* were found together with those of *S. haematobium* in the urine of a human patient. By laboratory passage he was able to obtain adults of both species from experimental infections in mice, however there was no definite evidence of hybridization In 1959 Pitchford described extensive infections of the cattle schistosome *S. mattheei* in man in the eastern Transvaal but these infections were always accompanied by either or both of the usual parasites of man in the area, *S. haematobium* and *S. mansoni*. There was some evidence of hybridization between *S. mattheei* and *S. haematobium* in these mixed infections and in 1961 Pitchford reported a case in which, by demonstrating the wide range of egg-shape in successive generations passaged through experimental animals, he provided very strong evidence of hybridization.

The first experimentally produced hybrids between terminal-spined schistosomes were achieved by Taylor (1970). In addition to repeating and confirming Le Roux's reciprocal crossing of the lateral spined species, *S. mansoni* and *S. rodhaini*, Taylor performed reciprocal crosses between *S. bovis* and *S. mattheei*. *S. bovis* females paired with *S. mattheei* males produced some viable eggs which, on passage through both parental intermediate hosts, yielded adult worms whose eggs were intermediate in shape between those of the parental species but the few eggs obtained from the cross *S. bovis* ♂ x *S. mattheei* ♀ were of such low viability that no successful snail infections were obtained. Taylor also produced viable crosses between males of a strain of *S. haematobium* from Nigeria with females of *S. bovis* and *S. mattheei* but a cross between male *S. haematobium* and female *S. bovis*, both of Iranian origin, was of very low viability. Repetition of the previous matings between *S. mansoni* ♂ x *S. mattheei* ♀ (Taylor *et al.*, 1969) yielded again parthenogenetic eggs which on passage gave rise to both male and female worms thus suggesting that in *S. mattheei* also the female is heterogametic. The mating *S. mansoni* ♂ x *S. bovis* ♀ gave rise to a few eggs of very low viability which did not establish infections in snails. Several of the hybrids resulting from the successful crosses in this series of experiments were maintained through a number of generations and their infectivity and pathogenicity to various vertebrate hosts were compared with those of the parental species (Taylor, 1971; Taylor and Andrews, 1973; Taylor *et al.*, 1973).

A report of successful hybridization between *S. mansoni* and *S. japonicum* has recently appeared in abstract form (Fan *et al.*, 1974). F_1 miracidia derived from the cross *S. mansoni* ♂ x *S. japonicum* ♀ are said to be infective to both of the parental host snails, *Biomphalaria glabrata* and *Oncomelania hupensis chiui* respectively, but those from the reciprocal cross are infective to the maternal host, *B. glabrata* only. Hybrid ova, miracidia and cercariae are all reported to resemble the maternal species in form and behaviour. These crosses were among those attempted by Vogel (1942) and although he reported the production of a few viable ova in the second alternative he attributed these to partheonogenesis, a point which Fan *et al.* specifically refute but without reasons.

Finally, Wright (1974) referred to the dual intermediate host behaviour of hybrid miracidia from the cross *S. mattheei* ♂ x *S. intercalatum* ♀ as evidence for the inheritance of a snail infectivity factor by schistosomes and Wright *et al.* (1974) and Southgate *et al.* (in press) described a focus of natural hybridization between *S. haematobium* and *S. intercalatum* in Cameroon. The main evidence in this case rested initially on the polymorphism of the eggs found and on the ability of the miracidia produced to develop in either of the parental host species. The experimental background to this study has provided much of the basis for the subsequent sections of this review.

RECIPROCITY OF INTERSPECIFIC PAIRINGS IN SCHISTOSOMES

Even in some of the interspecific pairings of schistosomes which do not result in hybridization there are apparent differences in the results of reciprocal matings. Thus, while females of *Schistosomatium douthitti* and *Schistosoma mattheei* will mature and produce parthenogenetic eggs when paired with males of *S. mansoni* the females of this species respond either very poorly or not at all to pairing with males of either of the other two (Short, 1948; Taylor, 1970). Vogel (1942) found that pairing of *S. mansoni* females with *S. japonicum* males resulted in the production of a few eggs but he achieved no success at all with the reverse mating, in contrast to the recent report of Fan *et al.* (1974) who claimed actual hybridization with both of these crosses. The crossing of *S. mansoni* and *S. rodhaini* appears to be equally successful in either combination of the two species (Le Roux, 1954a; Taylor, 1970) but so far no comparable results are forthcoming from the terminal spined schistosomes. In only one of Taylor's (1970) experiments did he succeed in obtaining reciprocal matings of a pair of terminal spined species and that was between *S. mattheei* and *S. bovis*. In this case the combination of *S. mattheei* ♂ x *S. bovis* ♀ resulted in enough eggs, albeit of low viability, to passage the hybrid and follow it through several generations but the reciprocal cross yielded eggs of such impaired viability that no snails were infected. Wright *et al.* (1974) found that the combination of *S. haematobium* (Cameroon) ♂ x *S. intercalatum* (Cameroon) ♀ is highly viable but the reverse mating produces few eggs, of very low viability. These combinations have now been repeated on several occasions and *S. haematobium* from two sources in Cameroon have been used, still with the same result. However, a recent cross between Cameroon *S. intercalatum* and *S. haematobium* from Cairo, Egypt has produced viable eggs in both combinations and the further results of these experiments are awaited. Mr. F. Frandsen informs us (private communication) that crosses between the Cameroon and Zaire strains of *S. intercalatum* are successful in both pairings although the viability of the eggs is low in both cases. Southgate *et al.* (in press) have obtained evidence to suggest that the cross *S. intercalatum* (Cameroon) ♂ x *S. haematobium* (Cameroon) ♀ is also non-viable in natural infections in man.

MORPHOLOGY OF THE EGGS OF HYBRID SCHISTOSOMES

Because egg shape and size are the main taxonomic characters in *Schistosoma*, and because in human infections the eggs are usually the only material available for study, it is not surprising that considerable attention has been given to this aspect of hybridization. However an important point concerning notation must be clarified before further discussion. The egg shells are the product of the vitelline cells of the female worm and they are shaped by the ootype of that female, thus the eggs from the initial cross between two species may contain a hybrid zygote but the shell is of maternal origin. While the developing embryo is of the F_1 generation the egg shell is of the P_1 generation. This point has led to some confusion in the literature where such eggs have frequently been referred to as F_1 with the result that those of subsequent generations are all moved forward by one. In this account the notation P_1 will be used to designate eggs derived from an initial cross between two species, the P_1 eggs hatch to release F_1 miracidia which in turn give rise to F_1 cercariae and adults and these produce the true F_1 eggs.

Evidence from some recent results (described below) suggests that the contained embryo may have some effect on the size of the egg but the basic shape of the shell must be under the influence of the genetic constitution of the female parent.

In all of the heterospecific matings which have resulted in the production of viable eggs all authors have reported that those eggs resemble the shape which is characteristic for the female parent, although occasionally some size differences have been noted, particularly in the case of parthenogentic eggs. It is in the descriptions of F_1 eggs where reports appear to vary somewhat. Thus both Le Roux (1954a) and Taylor (1970) found that the F_1 eggs of *S. mansoni* x *S. rodhaini* hybrids in either of the reciprocal matings were intermediate in shape between those of the two parental species but in some of the crosses between terminal spined species Taylor's results were less consistent. In the F_1 hybrid (F_2 in Taylor's notation) between *S. mattheei* ♂ x *S. bovis* ♀ the eggs showed a range of shapes through those of the two parental species and similar results were obtained from the F_1 hybrid *S. haematobium* (Nigeria) ♂ x *S. bovis* ♀ but in the cross *S. haematobium* (Nigeria) ♂ x *S. mattheei* ♀, although the P_1 eggs resembled those of the female parent the F_1 generation produced eggs resembling those of the male parent, *S. haematobium*, both in shape and size. In the F_2 generation from this cross the eggs continued to resemble *S. haematobium* in shape but the size was a little larger and intermediate between that of the two parental species. In the F_2 generations from the other crosses the polymorphism of the eggs was somewhat increased.

Pitchford (1961) passaged his suspected hybrid between *S. haematobium* and *S. mattheei* through several generations in rodents and recorded an apparent alternation of egg shapes in successive generations. The eggs originally isolated from a human infection were of *S. mattheei* shape while those from the first generation in *Mastomys* were somewhat intermediate but more like *S. haematobium*. The second generation was once more much like *S. mattheei* but a little shorter and the third generation was again like the first. In the fourth generation the range in shape was very wide covering both parental species but by the fifth and subsequent generations in *Mastomys* there appeared to have been a complete reversion to *S. mattheei* (Pitchford, 1965). Southgate *et al.* (in press) described the wide range of egg shapes seen in urine samples from children carrying hybrid infections of *S. haematobium* and *S. intercalatum* in Cameroon. By plotting cumulative size frequency curves on probability paper it was possible to show that the characteristics of these samples from natural infections differed from those of both of the parental species as well as from a simple mixture of the eggs of the parental species. Not only did the curve for the hybrid material lack the characteristic "step" which occurs in the curve for a bi-modal mixture of

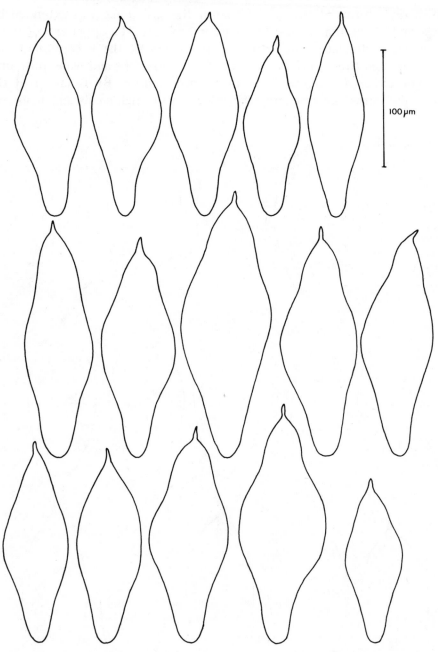

Fig. 1. Camera lucida drawings of viable P_1 eggs from the liver of a hamster infected with male *S. haematobium* (Cairo) and female *S. intercalatum* (Edea).

two distinct forms (Harding, 1949) but the size range was extended both below and above that of the two parental species. The upper end of the size range was particularly interesting in that many of the exceptionally large eggs resembled those of *S. bovis* in both size and shape and were quite unlike those of either *S. haematobium* or *S. intercalatum*. By isolation of these "*bovis*-like" eggs and passaging the infection through snails and hamsters it

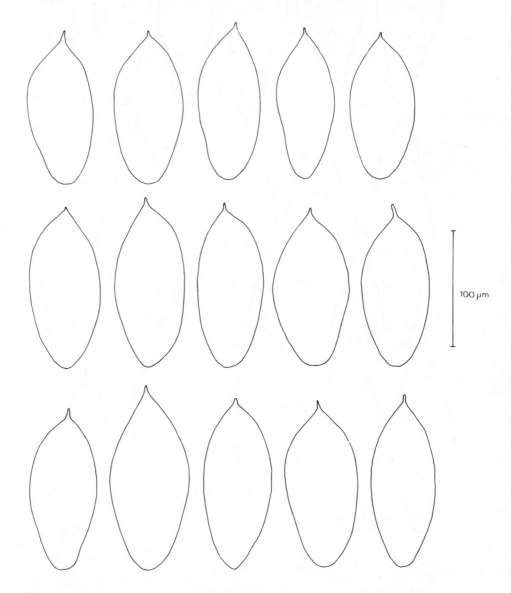

Fig. 2. Camera lucida drawings of viable P_1 eggs from the liver of a hamster infected with male *S. intercalatum* (Edea) and female *S. haematobium* (Cairo).

was shown that they gave rise to adult worms which produced eggs of size and shape throughout the hybrid range, thus confirming that the exceptional eggs were part of the hybrid series and did not represent an additional infection with a bovine parasite. It is interesting to note that in Pitchford's (1959) account of mixed infections of *S. mattheei* and *S. haematobium* in man in South Africa he mentioned the occurrence of some "*bovis*-like" eggs and it may be that these too were extreme forms in a hybrid series.

The results of our experimental crosses between *S. haematobium* and *S. intercalatum* confirm the general observations with respect to the P_1 generation in that the viable eggs resemble those of the maternal species in shape. Figs 1 & 2 illustrate eggs recovered from hamster livers for the reciprocal crosses between *S. haematobium* (Cairo) and *S. intercalatum* (Edea) (the only combination which yielded viable eggs in both combinations). However, from the cumulative size-frequency curves (Fig. 3)

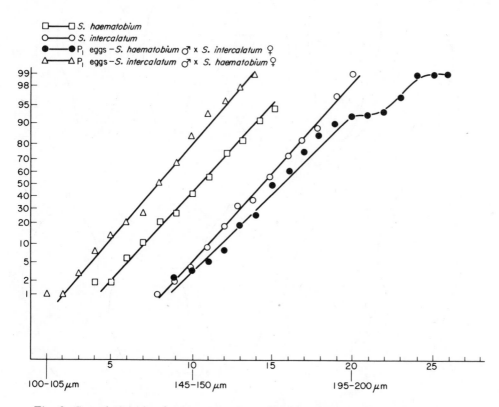

Fig. 3. Cumulative size-frequency curves of viable eggs from hamster livers of *S. haematobium* (Cairo), *S. intercalatum* (Edea) and the reciprocal crosses between them. Eggs resulting from the cross *S. haematobium* ♂ x *S. intercalatum* ♀ tend to be slightly larger than those of *S. intercalatum* while those resulting from the reciprocal mating tend to be smaller than those of the maternal species.

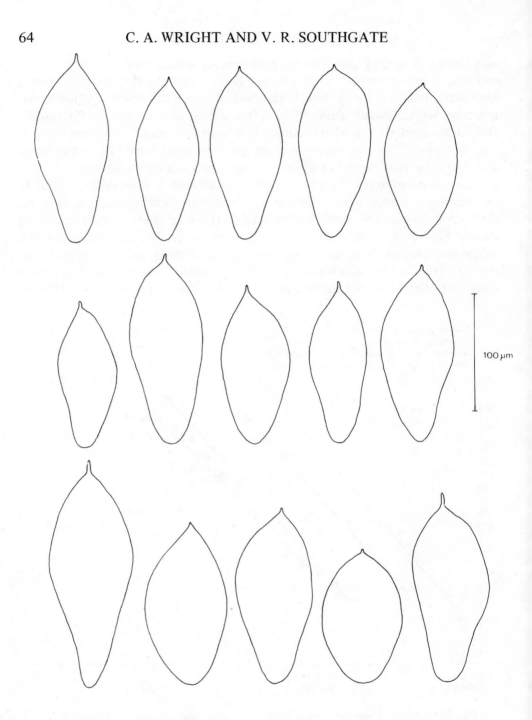

Fig. 4. Camera lucida drawings of viable F_1 eggs from the liver of a hamster carrying F_1 worms from the cross *S. haematobium* (Nyombe) ♂ x *S. intercalatum* (Edea) ♀

it can be seen that the eggs from these cross-matings tend to differ slightly in size from those of the parental species, those produced by the *S. intercalatum* ♂ x *S. haematobium* ♀ cross are smaller than those of *S. haematobium* while in the reverse pairing the eggs are slightly larger than those of *S. intercalatum*. The only material for suitable analysis at the F_1 generation as yet available is from the cross *S. haematobium* (Nyombe) ♂ x *S. intercalatum* (Edea) ♀. Eggs from these worms (Fig. 4) show a range of variation in size and shape which encompasses that of the two parental species (Southgate *et al.*, in press) and the size frequency graph for the hybrid eggs (Fig. 5) lies between the lines for the parental species, tending towards that for *S. intercalatum*. The irregularities at the lower end of the curve are probably due to the paucity of small eggs in the sample and it should be noted that there is no "step" in the graph in the region of overlap between the size ranges of the parental species, nor is there an extension at the upper end of the graph comparable to that seen in the natural hybrid

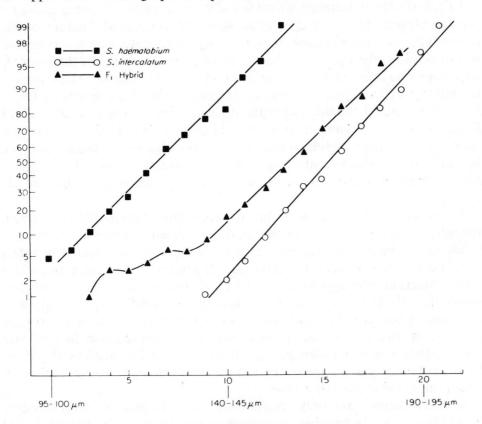

Fig. 5. Cumulative size-frequency curves for viable eggs from hamster livers of *S. haematobium* (Nyombe), *S. intercalatum* (Edea) and the F_1 hybrid from the cross *S. haematobium* (Nyombe) ♂ x *S. intercalatum* (Edea) ♀

samples. It is probable that the exceptionally large "*bovis*-like" eggs in the natural hybrid series are the result of back-crossing with one of the parental species. Possible evidence to support this idea has been forthcoming from one cross between *S. haematobium* (Nyombe) ♂ x *S. intercalatum* ♀. Previous experience had suggested that the schistosome infections at Nyombe were due to pure *S. haematobium* since both egg-morphology and intermediate host infectivity accorded with that species. Thus, when a fresh sample of eggs was received in London from Nyombe, single miracidial infections of snails were set up without prior examination of the material, and it was with some surprise that in a subsequent P_1 cross some "*bovis*-like" eggs were recovered. On checking the preserved portion of the original sample it was found that a hybrid range of eggs was present and that the male parent was probably not, therefore, pure *S. haematobium*.

The cross *S. intercalatum* ♂ x *S. haematobium* ♀ has proved to be not viable with either of the maternal parasite strains from Cameroon (Nyombe and Barombi Mbo) although with the Cairo strain plenty of viable eggs have been produced. There appears to be some variation in the nature of the non-viability of these crosses. In some only malformed eggs are produced and sometimes, the egg shape appears more or less normal but the contents are disorganised, in others, the eggs and their contained larvae appear normal but fail to hatch and in a very few cases miracidia have been produced. Of 10 *B. wrighti* exposed to such miracidia, derived from a cross with a female of *S. haematobium* (Nyombe), only two became infected and the cercariae from these yielded no adult worms in hamsters which were exposed to them. In an earlier experiment involving the Barombi Mbo strain of *S. haematobium* a single stunted male worm was recovered (Wright *et al.*, 1974).

In crosses involving female *S. haematobium* from Barombi Mbo, in which the intra-uterine eggs appear normal in shape but with disorganised contents, it has been found that eggs recovered from the livers of infected hamsters show no increase in size over those in the uteri of the females. In normal viable infections the eggs found in the host's tissues are usually about 20% longer than those *in utero* and the lack of any such difference in non-viable eggs suggest that it is the contained larvae which may be responsible for the increase. If this is the case it may provide an explanation for the size discrepancies noted between P_1 eggs from interspecific matings and those from the female parents in conspecific parings, although the mechanism by which this could occur is not clear.

S. intercalatum is the only species of African terminal spined schistosome in which the eggs, in histological sections of host tissue, stain red with carbol fuchsin used in the Ziehl-Neelsen technique (Becquet 1967). Southgate *et al.* (in press) reported that P_1 eggs produced by *S. intercalatum* females paired with *S. haematobium* males were, as would be expected, Ziehl-positive, but hamster tissues containing eggs derived from laboratory passage of natural hybrid infections showed both Ziehl-positive and negative eggs together. In this material there was a preponderance of eggs which failed to retain the stain and it was suggested that this might be due either to the presence of excess *S. haematobium* in the original sample or possibly to the recessive nature of the factors controlling the Ziehl-positive composition of the *S. intercalatum* egg shell. Initial attempts to continue this study in experimental hybrids failed, consequently particular care was taken to control subsequent observations. Although the majority of P_1 eggs produced by *S. intercalatum* ♀ paired with *S. haematobium* ♂ are Ziehl-positive there appear to be a small number which fail to retain the stain and this has also been noted in pure *S. intercalatum* from Cameroon. Sections of hamster tissues containing eggs derived from F_1 hybrids of which the male parent was *S. haematobium* from Barombi Mbo showed approximately equal numbers of positive and negative eggs while in the corresponding hybrid from male *S. haematobium* (Nyombe) there are more negative eggs than positive. These results suggest that, as with several other characters, the pattern of inheritance by the F_1 hybrid is dependent upon the paternal strain of *S. haematobium*.

INTERMEDIATE HOST INFECTIVITY OF HYBRID SCHISTOSOMES

One of the characteristics of the schistosomes is their high level of intermediate host restriction. All of the molluscan hosts for the African schistosome parasites of man and domestic animals develop in basommatophoran pulmonates of the family Planorbidae. The species of parasites with lateral spines on their eggs (*S. mansoni* and *S. rodhaini*) use snails of the genus *Biomphalaria* and those with terminal spines (*S. haematobium, S. bovis, S. mattheei, S. intercalatum* and *S. leiperi*) develop in species of *Bulinus*. Both of these snail genera are divided into a number of species groups and most of the schistosome parasites are restricted to one group or another. The divisions within *Biomphalaria* are of less significance in that *S. mansoni* is not so markedly specific in its host requirements but the five groups of *Bulinus* are of considerable relevance to the terminal spined species. These groups are *B. africanus, B. truncatus, B. tropicus, B. forskali* and *B. reticulatus.* The *B. tropicus* group need not be considered further here because none of its members act as hosts for any of the parasites under discussion, in fact it is only within the past year that the role of this group as hosts for *S. margrebowiei* has been discovered (Dr. R.J. Pitchford, private communication). The *B. reticulatus* group consists of a few probably "relic" species of which one, *B. wrighti*, is unique in that it is able to act as host for all known terminal-spined schistosomes and this has proved a useful asset in the establishment of various parasites in laboratory culture. The remaining three groups all have members which serve as hosts for some schistosomes but the pattern of host restriction varies, some of the parasite species have strains restricted to certain species within a group or even to particular populations of a snail species, while others have a much wider spectrum of host utilisation. A full account of the finer points of this phenomenon is not appropriate to this review but it is important to establish the broad principles because they are fundamental to one of the most interesting consequences of hybridization of the parasites.

Le Roux's (1954a) successful crossing of *S. mansoni* and *S. rodhaini* resulted in hybrids which were infective to *Biomphalaria alexandrina*, a species which had not previously been infected with *S. rodhaini*, and *B. glabrata* proved to be more susceptible to the hybrids than to *S. rodhaini*. Taylor's (1970) crosses between the same two species yielded similar results with increased infectivity for *B. glabrata* in the hybrid derived from the *S. rodhaini* female and enhanced infectivity for *B. pfeifferi* and *B. sudanica* in the reciprocal mating. These results are fairly conclusive, nevertheless they leave some room for speculation in that other authors have presented different pictures of the snail host range for *S. rodhaini*. Howaldt and Pitchford (1963) found that both *B. glabrata* and *B. pfeifferi* were susceptible to this species and Saoud (1966), whose experiments were more extensive, concluded that different strains of the parasite probably have different snail host ranges.

It is in the restricted relationships between terminal spined parasites and their bulinid hosts that the evidence is more convincing. Nothing can be deduced from Pitchford's (1961) suggestion of crossing between *S. mattheei* and *S. haematobium* in South Africa because both parasites in that area use the same snail hosts, members of the *B. africanus* group. However, some of Taylor's (1970) experimental results are interesting in that he succeeded in producing hybrids between parasites with hosts usually considered to be mutually exclusive. Thus the offspring of the cross *S. mattheei* ♂ x *S. bovis* ♀ developed in both the *B. africanus* group snails used by *S. mattheei* and in the *B. truncatus* snails used by *S. bovis*. Again an element of doubt is introduced here by Howaldt and Armstrong's (1969) report that each of these parental species could develop in the normal host for the other but attempts in our own laboratory to repeat this have so far failed. Taylor's cross between a Nigerian strain of *S. haematobium* and the Iranian *S. bovis* became established in both the *africanus* group hosts for the male parent and those of the *truncatus* group used by the female parent but his hybrid between the Nigerian *S. haematobium* and *S. mattheei* was unusual in that although both of the parental species use *africanus* group snails successful hybrid infections were only established in the hosts for the maternal *S. mattheei*, no more than one specimen of the paternal host becoming infected.

The recent experiments involving the lower Guinea strain of *S. intercalatum* have the advantage that the intermediate host range of this parasite has probably been more extensively investigated than any other. Wright *et al.* (1972) exposed over 4,000 snails to this strain of parasite and, with one aberrant exception, it was shown to develop exclusively in members of the *B. forskali* and *B. reticulatus* groups. Since that report at least as many snails again have been exposed and, without exception, the original results have been confirmed and a new record, *B. crystallinus* (*B. forskali* group) from Angola has been added to the list of those susceptible to infection. In the experiments briefly reported by Wright (1974) the progeny of the cross *S. mattheei* ♂ x *S. intercalatum* ♀ were equally infective to the paternal *africanus* group and maternal *forskali* group snails. This infectivity persisted through to the F_3 generation even when the parasite was cycled solely through the paternal host in each generation and it was not until F_4 that infectivity to the original maternal hosts was apparently lost. When the natural focus of hybridization between *S. haematobium* and *S. intercalatum* was first suspected in Loum, snail infection experiments showed that miracidia hatched from the polymorphic eggs obtained in urine samples were equally infective to both the *B. truncatus* group hosts for *S. haematobium* and to *B. forskali* group snails. This did not eliminate the possibility of a simple mixed infection so the cercariae from the two snail groups were passaged separately through hamsters and in the next cycle the dual infectivity was still retained in both lines, thus confirming the presence of hybrids in the original infection (Wright *et al.*, 1974; Southgate *et al.*, in press).

The three strains of *S. haematobium* which we have used for experimental crosses are of the type which develop in *B. truncatus* group snails. All of these strains are also likely to develop in certain members of the *B. forskali* group (*B. bavayi*, *B. beccarii*, *B. cernicus*, *B. senegalensis* and *B. camerunensis*) therefore the only members of this group which have been used for checking hybrid infectivity are those in which *S. haematobium* is not known normally to develop (*B. forskali*, *B. scalaris* and *B. crystallinus*). Each of the parental strains of *S. haematobium* has been tested against these species with uniformly negative outcome and Table 1 gives the overall infections results of these strains in *B. truncatus* group snails (*B. truncatus* and *B. rohlfsi* of various origins). Table 2 summarises the results of snail infection experiments with F_1 hybrid miracidia from crosses in which the male parents were from each of the *S. haematobium* strains.

Table 1
Overall infection results of the three parental strains of *S. haematobium* in *B. truncatus* group snails

Strain of *S. haematobium*	No. snails exposed	No. surviving prepatent period	No. infected	% survivors infected	mean prepatent period (days)
Barombi Mbo, Cameroon	280	244	65	26.6	35
Nyombe, Cameroon	130	128	22	17.2	33
Cairo, Egypt	175	163	61	37.5	33

Table 2
Summarised results of snail infection experiments with F_1 hybrid miracidia derived from crosses of female *S. intercalatum* with males of three strains of *S. haematobium* (Barombi Mbo, Cameroon; Nyombe, Cameroon and Cairo, Egypt)

Snail group	No. exposed	No. surviving prepatent period	No. infected	% survivors infected	Mean prepatent period (days)
F_1 *S. haematobium* Barombi Mbo ♂ x *S. intercalatum* Edea ♀					
B. forskali	185	135	34	25.2	31
B. truncatus	175	145	55	37.9	32
B. wrighti	50	37	8	21.6	33
F_1 *S. haematobium* Nyombe ♂ x *S. intercalatum* Edea ♀					
B. forskali	150	67	7	10.5	26
B. truncatus	100	84	12	14.3	26
B. wrighti	150	142	66	46.5	26
F_1 *S. haematobium* Cairo ♂ x *S. intercalatum* Edea ♀					
B. forskali	80	60	14	23.4	28
B. truncatus	25	25	8	32.0	26
B. wrighti	80	80	29	36.2	22

These results show clearly the dual infectivity of the hybrid parasites for each of the parental snail host groups. The percentage infection rates achieved in paternal (*B. truncatus*) hosts are roughly similar to those in Table 1 for the strains of *S. haematobium* in snails of the same group but the results for *B. forskali* group snails are markedly lower than those normally obtained for *S. intercalatum* in the same hosts (Wright *et al.*, 1972; Frandsen, 1975). The figures for the prepatent periods suggest that in the cross with *S. haematobium* from Barombi Mbo the time is closer to that for the paternal species while in the other two crosses the times are nearer to that for *S. intercalatum* (22 days). However, the results for the two last crosses were obtained during the recent hot summer when temperatures in the aquarium room rose well above the normal control level of 25°C for long periods, reaching a peak of 32°C, and consequently the figures cannot be usefully compared.

The drop in infectivity for *B. forskali* group snails is evidence of some impairment of the viability of F_1 miracidia in these crosses but this appears to be offset by the undiminished infectivity for the paternal intermediate hosts, a point which may well have significance in the development of the natural focus of hybridization at Loum (Southgate *et al.*, in press).

Preliminary results of snail infection experiments using F_2 miracidia of the *S. haematobium* (Nyombe) ♂ x *S. intercalatum* (Edea) ♀ cross are given in Table 3. Unfortunately the numbers of snails used are small and the

Table 3

Snail infection experiments with F_2 miracidia derived from the cross *S. haematobium* (Nyombe) ♂ x *S. intercalatum* (Edea) ♀

Snail group	No. exposed	No. surviving prepatent period	No. infected	% survivors infected	Mean prepatent period (days)
B. forskali	75	19	7	37	27
B. truncatus	75	48	11	23	27
B. wrighti	50	23	9	35	27

figures for the percentage infection rates of survivors are not helpful because of the high mortality of the snails during the prepatent period. The high death rates may be due to infectivity of the parasites or equally to the condition of the snails at the time of exposure. The small numbers used are a result of the prolonged period of overheating of the aquarium room during which there was a marked reduction in breeding in the snail colonies. However during the period of this experiment the temperature of the room had returned to its normal controlled level of 25°C and the prepatent period of 27 days is therefore comparable with that of 33 days for *S. haematobium* (Nyombe) (Table 1) and 22 days for *S. intercalatum* (Edea).

When these experiments were originally designed it was intended that by exposing snails of both parental host groups, together with *B. wrighti*, to infection by F_2 miracidia some useful data on inheritance of infectivity might be obtained. It was hoped that if segregation of the characters determining infectivity occurred it might be detected in differential infection rates in the host groups. Each of the parental host species should be susceptible to its own parasite plus the hybrid while *B. wrighti* is susceptible to both parental parasite species as well as the hybrid. Not only are the present results totally inadequate but the reduced infectivity of the F_1 hybrid parasite to *S. intercalatum* snail hosts is likely to make the matter much more complicated than was originally thought.

Perhaps the most interesting feature of this hybrid infectivity is the light which it sheds on the host parasite relationship between trematodes and their molluscan hosts (Wright, 1974). It demonstrates clearly the inheritance of factors which enable the parasite larvae to evade the innate responses of the molluscs to invasive foreign bodies. This places more emphasis on the role of the parasites in establishing successful infections in snails whereas in the past the question of snail susceptibility has been accorded more attention. If *S. intercalatum* miracidia penetrate snails of the *B. truncatus* group they survive for a very brief period and are then encapsulated by concentric layers of the hosts' amoebocytes but the hybrid larvae inherit from their male parent some characteristic which enables them to continue successful development in *B. truncatus* group snails and to achieve infection rates comparable with those of the paternal species.

BEHAVIOUR OF HYBRID CERCARIAE

No information is forthcoming on behavioural changes in larval stages of hybrid schistosomes. Fan *et al.* (1974) merely report that the miracidia and cercariae derived from their crosses between *S. mansoni* and *S. japonicum* resemble the maternal species in form and behaviour. Neither Le Roux (1954a) nor Taylor (1970) make any mention of the diurnal rhythm of cercerial emergence in their crosses between *S. mansoni* and *S. rodhaini* despite the fact that the two parental species have distinctive periodicity in this respect. Wright *et al.* (1972) showed that the cercariae of *S. intercalatum* have two behavioural characteristics not yet seen in other species of African schistosomes, they exhibit a very marked predilection for the surface film and they have a strong tendency to form tightly knit aggregations in response to thermal stimuli.

Experimental attempts to quantify the vertical distribution of cercariae of *S. haematobium, S. intercalatum* and their hybrid have been carried out in a cell 8 cms high 2.5 cms wide and 0.5 cms thick. Known numbers of larvae are introduced into the cell, left undisturbed for 30 minutes and then photographed using a flash source beneath the cell. Four equal (2cm) depth

Table 4

Depth distribution of cercaria of *S. haematobium*, Nyombe, Cameroon, *S. intercalatum*. Edea, Cameroon and their F_1 hybrid, zone A is the bottom and zone D the top of the cell

		A	B	C	D
S. haematobium, Nyombe,	1	8.4	21.6	6.6	63.4
	2	15.0	15.0	22.5	47.5
	3	6.7	10.0	18.3	65.0
	Mean	10.0	15.8	15.8	58.6
S. intercalatum, Edea.	1	0	1.1	6.4	92.5
	2	0	3.1	1.6	95.3
	3	0	2.1	1.1	96.8
	Mean	0	2.1	3.0	94.8
F_1 Hybrid *S. haematobium* Nyombe ♂ x	1	13.7	11.6	14.3	61.0
S. intercalatum Edea ♀	2	13.1	18.3	21.8	46.8
	3	2.8	5.6	9.5	82.1
	4	10.1	8.8	11.1	70.0
	5	8.3	7.3	9.3	75.1
	Mean	9.5	10.3	13.2	67.0

zones from A (bottom) to D (top) are marked on the photographs and the cercariae in each zone are counted and expressed as a percentage of the total. Table 4 sets out the results of a series of such experiments using a strain of *S. haematobium* from Nyombe, Cameroon, *S. intercalatum*, Edea, Cameroon and F_1 cercariae from their hybrid (*S. haematobium* ♂ x *S. intercalatum* ♀). It is apparent in this case that the behaviour of the hybrid cercariae with respect to depth distribution more closely resembles that of *S. haematobium* than *S. intercalatum*. However, similar experiments involving F_1 hybrid cercariae from the cross *S. haematobium* (Cairo) ♂ x *S. intercalatum* (Edea) ♀ showed that 90.9% of the cercariae were concentrated in the upper zone (D) with 9.1% in zone C. In this cross, therefore, the hybrid behaviour pattern resembles that of *S. intercalatum*. Although comparable experiments were not made using the cross *S. haematobium* (Barombi Mbo) ♂ x *S. intercalatum* (Edea) ♀ it was noted that the behaviour of these F_1 cercariae also resembled that of *S. intercalatum*.

Tests on the aggregation response to thermal stimuli have also been carried out. The mechanism of this aggregation has been examined at the fine structure level and the histological and histochemical observations, suggesting that it is secretion from the post-acetabular glands which causes adhesion (Wright *et al.*, 1972), have been confirmed. More detailed experiments on the thermal stimulus have shown that at water temperatures between 20°C and 30°C increases of as little as 0.5°C at a point are sufficient to induce aggregation. No aggregation has been seen in cercariae of *S. haematobium* of any of the three strains used in these experiments but the larvae of *S. intercalatum* Edea respond strongly. The tendency to aggregate occurs readily in F_1 hybrid cercariae resulting from crosses between the Barombi Mbo and Cairo strains of *S. haematobium* and *S. intercalatum* but cannot be induced in F_1 cercariae of the cross with Nyombe *S. haematobium*. Aggregation also occurs in F_1 cercariae of the cross *S. mattheei* ♂ x *S. intercalatum* ♀.

These results show that inheritance by hybrids of the behavioural traits of *S. intercalatum* cercariae depend upon the strain of *S. haematobium* acting as paternal parent. In the cross with *S. haematobium* from Nyombe the behaviour patterns of *S. intercalatum* are suppressed in the hybrid larvae but are present in those derived from crosses with the Barombi Mbo and Cairo strains of *S. haematobium*.

DEFINITIVE HOST INFECTIVITY OF HYBRID SCHISTOSOMES

In all of Taylor's (1970) cross-matings of schistosomes, in both the terminal spined and lateral spined species complexes, delayed maturation of the female worms occurred. In some cases the delay corresponded to the normal period for the species to which the male worms belonged but in others it was prolonged beyond the normal time for either species. In those pairings which resulted in subsequent generations most showed a maturation of the F_1 hybrids similar to that of the original maternal species but in others the period was slower. Although Taylor (1970) gives percentage worm returns (the number of adult worms recovered from an experimental animal expressed as a percentage of the number of cercariae to which the animal was exposed; used as an index of the infectivity of the cercariae for the animal concerned) for several of his F_1 hybrids and in some cases for F_2 generations also, these are not compared with similar figures for the parental species. Nevertheless some of these worm returns for hybrids appear to be very high and suggest enhanced success of the hybrid cercariae. In subsequent studies (Taylor and Andrews, 1973), using F_3 and F_4 generation hybrids, the worm return figures in hamsters are compared with those of the parental species. In those crosses involving *S. mattheei* with either *S. bovis* or *S. haematobium* the hybrid returns are almost exactly intermediate between those for the original parental species but in the cross *S. rodhaini* ♂ x *S.*

mansoni ♀ the infectivity of the F_4 hybrid cercariae appears to be considerably greater than that of either of the parental species or the F_4 generation of the reciprocal cross. Further results, based upon experiments using baboons (Taylor *et al.*, 1973), were complicated by the fact that some of the parental species (*S. rodhaini* and *S. bovis*) failed to develop in these hosts. Unfortunately the precise genetic constitution of an F_3 and F_4 hybrid is difficult to determine due to possible segregation and backcrossing in preceding generations and direct comparisons of these results with others is not therefore possible.

In our recent experimental crosses between *S. haematobium* (Nyombe) ♂ x *S. intercalatum* (Edea) ♀ there does not appear to have been any significant delay in maturation of the female worms in the P_1 generation. Because the main object of the initial crosses was to provide sufficient eggs for snail infection experiments, the earliest time for which we have data on the parasites is 64 days after infection of the hamster. In this animal there were 35 pairs of worms and the mean length of the *S. haematobium* males was 12.3 mm, that of the *S. intercalatum* females 12.1 mm and the mean uterine egg count was 33.5 with 97% of the females gravid. Comparison with the data on maturation of both parental species in Table 5 suggests that the growth of the male worms was somewhat enhanced, that of the females slightly decreased, the percentage gravid slightly above the mean and the uterine egg count about double that in *S. intercalatum* of comparable age. The F_1 parasites derived from this cross show (Table 5) accelerated growth of the males exceeding that of either parental species but the females lag behind the maternal species until the 70th day when they are roughly equal in size to those of *S. intercalatum*. At 50 days both the uterine egg count of the F_1 females and the percentage which are gravid are slightly lower than the figures for *S. intercalatum* but by 60 and 70 days the hybrids are well ahead, particularly in the uterine egg count. It would be premature to presume that egg productivity per adult female was similarly enhanced nevertheless it seems highly likely that this may prove to be the case. An index of maturation for schistosome species, which has proved to be useful in earlier studies, is the "cross-over point", the age at which female worms equal male worms in length (in most species of *Schistosoma* the females are much smaller than the males in the early stages of development but in the mature state they attain considerably greater body length). In the Cameroon strain of *S. intercalatum* this point is reached at about 49 days while in *S. haematobium* the period is about 80-85 days. In the F_1 hybrid between Cameroon strains of the two species the "cross-over point" is achieved at about 54 days, slightly later than that for the maternal species but very much earlier than for *S. haematobium*.

The worm return results for the F_1 hybrid show a marked increase over

Table 5*

Maturation of S. intercalatum, S. haematobium and the F₁ hybrid S. haematobium ♂ x S. intercalatum ♀ in hamsters.

Parasite species	Male worms Mean length			Female worms Mean length			Mean uterine egg-count			% gravid females		
	50	60	70	50	60	70	50	60	70	50	60	70
S. intercalatum (Edea)	9.5	10.5	12.0	10.1	14.2	16.1	12.1	12.4	19.1	74.5	91.3	84.1
S. haematobium (Nyombe)	8.9	8.4	10.8	5.5	9.6	13.5	0	0	0	0	0	0
S. haematobium (Average of 4 strains)	8.0	9.5	11.0	4.0	7.5	9.0	0	9.0	15.0	0	24.0	59.0
S. haematobium ♂ x S. intercalatum ♀) F₁	10.1	11.5	14.8	8.6	12.8	16.7	10.7	22.0	27.6	51.9	92.1	98.9

* Data for S. intercalatum from Wright et al. (1972) and for the average of four strains of S. haematobium from Wright and Knowles (1972). Figures for S. intercalatum and the F₁ hybrid based upon five hamsters for each ten day period, those for S. haematobium (Nyombe) on one hamster each and the average for the four strains of S. haematobium on five animals for each strain for each period.

those for either of the parental species in hamsters. The mean figure for *S. intercalatum* is 17.3% (Wright *et al.*, 1972) but the figures for the Nyombe strain of *S. haematobium* which are available are so low that they are probably unrealistic. Worm returns for six other strains of *S. haematobium* in hamsters range from 17.8% (Dezful, Iran) to 36.4% (Pokoase, Ghana) with an average of 25.9% (Wright and Bennett, 1967, a and b; Wright and Knowles, 1972). The mean figure for 15 hamsters exposed to the F_1 hybrid is 47.5% with a range from 18.5% to 86%.

The picture that emerges so far is of an F_1 hybrid which tends towards its maternal species in the rapidity of its development but is three times as infective to hamsters as *S. intercalatum* and about twice as infective as the average *S. haematobium*. The uterine egg counts also suggest that the potential egg-output of the hybrid may be greater than that of either of the parental species.

ISOENZYMES OF HYBRID SCHISTOSOMES

Several reports of isoenzymes in schistosomes have been published (Coles, 1970 and 1971a and b; Wright *et al.*, 1972; Southgate and Knowles, 1975). Our preliminary studies on the enzymes of *S. haematobium*, *S. intercalatum* and their hybrid employed a thin-layer starch gel technique and the results were unsatisfactory for useful analysis. More recently we have employed the method of isoelectric focusing and although the work is still in its early stages the results are more promising (Ross, in press). A preliminary examination of nine systems was made—lactate, malate, glutamate, galactose, succinate and glucose 6—phosphate dehydrogenases, acid and alkaline phosphatases and non-specific esterases. Of these only the lactate (LDH) and malate (MDH) dehydrogenases and acid phosphatases gave results which seemed to merit further immediate study. The last two of these systems proved of value in work on strains of *S. bovis* (Southgate and Knowles, 1975) but in the *S. haematobium* x *S. intercalatum* hybrid study they have not been pursued because of the close similarity in the patterns of the two parental species. It is possible that a group of three bands in the region pH 5.7-6.3 in the MDH pattern may be of value when they are more clearly resolved by use of ampholines selected for this pH range. The LDH system which failed to contribute much to the *S. bovis* problem has shown more promise when applied to the current hybrid study.

Eleven LDH fractions have been resolved in extracts from male *S. haematobium* (Nyombe) and only nine in the same species from Cairo. The females of these two strains have so far yielded only five and two bands respectively, the deficiency in the pattern of the females from Cairo can probably be attributed simply to low concentration. Two of the five

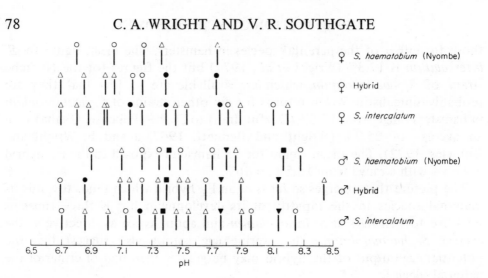

Fig. 6. Diagrammatic representation of the lactate dehydrogenase (LDH) isoenzymes separated by isoelectric focusing in acrylamide gel, of *S. haematobium* (Nyombe), *S. intercalatum* (Edea) and the F_1 hybrid from the cross *S. haematobium* (Nyombe) ♂ x *S. intercalatum* (Edea) ♀ The upper three sets show patterns for female worms, the lower three for males. Symbols above the lines indicate the intensity of the fractions represented:- open circles—faint; open triangles— +; filled circles— ++; filled squares— +++; inverted filled triangles— ++++.

fractions in the female *S. haematobium* (Nyombe) are not represented in the eleven present in the males. Both male and female *S. intercalatum* (Edea) show fifteen LDH fractions but not all of these appear to be identical in the two sexes. It is premature to draw conclusions concerning the significance of apparent differences in relative concentration and slight differences in isoelectric point of these fractions but the greater complexity of the pattern in *S. intercalatum* is obvious when compared to that of *S. haematobium*. At present we allow a tolerance of 0.05 pH units in determining whether or not certain fractions in different patterns correspond but the validity of this tolerance remains to be established.

The patterns obtained from *S. haematobium* (Nyombe), *S. intercalatum* (Edea) and their F_1 hybrid are illustrated in Fig. 6. F_1 hybrid males give fourteen LDH fractions of which probably ten are in common with those of the *S. haematobium* males and twelve correspond to twelve of the fifteen in *S. intercalatum* males. Three of the *S. intercalatum* male fractions are clearly absent from the hybrid male pattern also one of the *S. haematobium* bands, but the hybrid has a distinctive band beyond the alkaline range of either of the parental species. F_1 hybrid females from the same cross have eight fractions, four of which correspond to four of the five in *S. haematobium* females and at least six of the hybrid fractions appear to correspond to six of the fifteen in female *S. intercalatum*. Although females of both parental species have a fraction at pH 6.81 there is no corresponding band in the female hybrid but it has a band at pH 6.86 not present in the females of either parental species but present in the male *S. intercalatum* and in the male hybrid. In general appearance the male F_1 hybrid pattern appears to have more in common with that of male *S. intercalatum* while the female F_1 hybrids give patterns more like those of female *S. haematobium* in that they lack many of the alkaline fractions of female *S. intercalatum*.

Further detailed study of more material is obviously essential, particularly the progeny from back-cross combinations. However, it is vital that hybrid material must be referred to the parental species at corresponding generations of passage in experimental animals. Coles (1971b) reported the loss of two fast-running (starch gel) MDH bands in *S. mansoni* on passage through mice and recently Ross (in press) has noted the disappearance of a group of MDH fractions in the extreme alkaline end of the pH range in a strain of *S. bovis* from Kenya after three passages in hamsters. Analysis of the inheritance of isoenzyme patterns in hybrid schistosomes is likely to prove complex enough without the addition of host-influenced factors to confuse the matter further.

DISCUSSION

The basic objective of most studies on hybridization of schistosomes has been elucidation of the taxonomic relationships within *Schistosoma*. At the species-group level Taylor (1970) has shown clearly that complete genetic isolation exists between the parasites with terminal-spined eggs and those with lateral spines. The production of a partially viable experimental cross between *S. mansoni* and *S. japonicum* (Fan *et al.*, 1974) suggests a closer relationship between these species than has been generally accepted. The report by Pao (quoted by Mao, 1962) of a schistosome belonging to the *S. mansoni* complex in wild rodents in south-west China may be relevant here. This parasite was said to use snails of the amnicolid prosobranch genus *Tricula* as intermediate hosts. Another species originally attributed to *Tricula* on Taiwan has since been shown to belong to *Oncomelania* (Davis, 1968) and this is the species used by Fan *et al.* as host for *S. japonicum* in their experiments. If the snail host for the *S. mansoni*-like parasite in China should also prove to be an oncomelaniid it might well support the evidence of the hybridisation experiments for a closer relationship between the lateral-spined schistosomes and *S. japonicum*.

Within the species complexes, Taylor's (1970) results show a high level of genetic compatibility between the two African species with lateral-spined eggs, *S. mansoni* and *S. rodhaini*. It is probable that differences in definitive hosts help to maintain the distinction between these two in nature, despite areas of overlap in their range and the use of similar snail hosts. In the terminal-spined group the relationships are more complicated. So far all of the interspecific matings which have been investigated experimentally appear to be at least partially successful but they range from the almost completely non-viable cross between the sympatric Iranian *S. haematobium* x *S. bovis* to the possibly reciprocal viability of the *S. haematobium* (Cairo) x *S. intercalatum* (Edea) cross reported in this paper. The moderate success of the cross between *S. bovis* (Iran) x *S. haematobium* (Nigeria) suggests that in addition to the separate definitive hosts of the two parasites some genetic mechanism has evolved to maintain the distinction between the two species in Iran.

The extent to which the results of hybridization experiments should influence current taxonomic usage at the species level is open to question. By all accepted criteria the failure of two sympatric species to interbreed is clear evidence that they are "good" species but with allopatric forms there is no easy answer. Do Frandsen's observations on the low viability of crosses between the Zaire and Lower Guinea strains of *S. intercalatum* mean that these two forms are less closely related than are the Lower Guinea strains of *S. intercalatum* and *S. haematobium* which yield viable one-way hybrids in nature? Or, is the Egyptian strain of *S. haematobium* more closely related to Lower Guinea *S. intercalatum* because of the reciprocal viability of the experimental cross? The only clear distinction between the two strains of *S. intercalatum* is that they use different snail intermediate hosts but in their morphology and behaviour they appear to be very similar. On the other hand not only does *S. haematobium* use different snail hosts from those of the Lower Guinea strain of *S. intercalatum* but there are also morphological and behavioural differences between the two. Although the evolutionary origins of parasites must be subject to a great deal of speculation it is probable that both *S. haematobium* and *S. intercalatum* originated from a common stock and that *S. haematobium* evolved as a parasite of the hominoid precursors of man in savannah areas (Wright, 1970) while *S. intercalatum* evolved as a parasite of forest-living primates (Wright *et al.*, 1972). Both of the species have undergone some degree of infra-specific differentiation by isolation of populations within their respective habitat types, but the isolation of the two major stocks has perhaps persisted for a very considerable period of time. By reason of their ecological separation they have diverged to become two distinctive forms without the evolution of genetical isolating mechanisms. Whether as a result these distinctive forms should be regarded as species or sub-species seems to be largely a matter of semantics. Perhaps a more practical point which has emerged from these observations on hybridization is the further illustration of genetic differences between populations of the same species. Differences in the reciprocal viability of crosses between the Lower Guinea strain of *S. intercalatum* and the Cameroon and Egyptian strains of *S. haematobium*, and differences in the inheritance of cercarial behaviour patterns and egg-shell staining characteristics, all serve to emphasize the need for caution in extrapolating from the results of studies on a parasite species in one part of its range to another (Wright, 1962).

Inheritance of intermediate host infectivity by hybrid schistosomes calls for some re-examination of the role of molluscan hosts in trematode speciation (Wright, 1960). The experimental evidence of Boray (1966) who produced a "new" strain of *Fasciola hepatica* in only two generations by passage through a species of *Lymnaea* which is not normally a host for the parasite and Saoud's (1965) demonstration of changes in an Egyptian strain of *Schistosoma mansoni* after 15 years of passage in a South American species of *Biomphalaria* are both suggestive of marked influences on the parasites by their snail hosts. Also if two closely related parasites have different molluscan host requirements there is less chance of them both becoming established in an area where only one or other of the hosts exists and they will thus be effectively isolated. However it is now apparent that where both molluscan hosts coexist and interbreeding of the parasites can occur intermediate host restriction will cease to be an effective isolating mechanism.

Where hybridization of *S. haematobium* and the ungulate parasite *S. mattheei* has occurred in South Africa the question of molluscan host restriction is not involved because both species develop in the same snails. Taylor (1970) has suggested that this situation may have arisen as the result of intensive livestock farming in the area, breaking down the ecological isolation between *S. mattheei* which probably evolved as a parasite of antelopes and the human *S. haematobium*. Southgate *et al.* (in press) have put forward a somewhat similar explanation for the focus of hybridization between *S. haematobium* and *S. intercalatum* at Loum in Cameroon. Here extensive forest clearance followed by large-scale agricultural development has made the streams suitable for colonization by the snail hosts for *S. haematobium* and this parasite has thus been able to become established in an area where previously only the forest species *S. intercalatum* existed. Since both species are parasites of man there has been no definitive host barrier to interbreeding and as we have shown the potential barrier of intermediate host restriction has broken down. Both of these examples appear to be the result of recent man-made alterations to the environment. Similar situations could arise by movements of definitive host populations or through natural environmental changes and it is possible that some of the contemporary strains of *Schistosoma* are derived from localised hybridization.

In North Africa and the Middle East *S. haematobium* develops in snails of the *B. truncatus* group while south of the Sahara it is the *B. africanus* group which act as hosts. Each of these forms of *S. haematobium* will not normally develop in the snail hosts used by the other and in West Africa where both forms occur this intermediate host restriction is generally maintained. In Ghana, however there are strains of the parasite which can utilise both snail host groups (Paperna, 1968). Comparison of two of these strains with *S. haematobium* from other areas has shown that they grow more rapidly, reach larger maximum size and produce about double the worm return in hamsters (Wright and Knowles, 1972). These characteristics, in conjunction with their dual intermediate host infectivity, are comparable with those of the F_1 *S. haematobium* x *S. intercalatum* cross described in this paper and are strongly suggestive of hybridization between the *B. truncatus* and *B. africanus* borne strains of *S. haematobium*. Another example which might be the result of hybridization is found in the Kenya strain of *S. bovis* which develops in nature in snails of the *B. truncatus*, *B. africanus* and *B. forskali* groups (Southgate and Knowles, in press). Although most of the characteristics of this strain conform to *S. bovis* such a broad intermediate host range is so far not known in any other African schistosome. Kenya could also be an area where a further problem might develop in the future. The Kenyan strain of *S. haematobium* is restricted to snail hosts of the *B. africanus* group, but snails of the *B. truncatus* group have recently been identified in the country over a wide area (Brown and Wright, 1974; Southgate and Knowles, 1975). These snails are susceptible to strains of *S. haematobium* which develop in *B. truncatus* group hosts in other areas (recent exposure of snails from Ahero to a Cairo strain of parasite resulted in infections in 81% of the survivors), and if such parasite strains are introduced to Kenya they could easily become established and interbreed with the local *B. africanus*-borne form.

In describing the focus of hybridization between *S. haematobium* and *S. intercalatum* at Loum in Cameroon, Southgate *et al.* (in press) drew attention to the way in which *S. haematobium* and the hybrid appeared to be replacing the endemic *S. intercalatum* in the five years since *S. haematobium* first appeared in the town. It was suggested that the hybrid, in addition to its ability to use either snail host species, shared with *S. haematobium* the advantage of urinary discharge of its eggs, thus more easily evading the basic level of sanitation in the town, and that *B. rohlfsi* being a larger snail than *B. forskali* is capable of producing greater numbers of cercariae. To these advantages can now be added the relatively greater infectivity of the hybrid for *B. rohlfsi*, the increased infectivity of hybrid cercariae relative to either of the parental species, the rapid maturation time of the hybrid parasites both in snails and hamsters (closer to *S. intercalatum* than *S. haematobium*) and potentially greater egg-production by the hybrid adults. So far the only deleterious character of the hybrid which we have been able to identify is its reduced infectivity to *B. forskali* relative to that of *S. intercalatum* but this is probably more than off-set by its advantages and will only serve to shift the balance between the parental species further in favour of *S. haematobium*. The probable outcome of this situation will be a new strain of *S. haematobium* in which will be retained the advantageous characteristics of the hybrid.

An account of a recent attempt to control transmission of *S. haematobium* at the small lake focus of Barombi Kotto in Cameroon (Duke and Moore, in prep. a and b) suggests that some of these observations are of more than academic interest. At this focus the most important snail host was *B. rohlfsi* with *B. camerunensis* playing a minor part in transmission. *B. camerunensis* is a member of the *B. forskali* group with limited susceptibility to local *S. haematobium* but, under experimental conditions, an excellent host for *S. intercalatum*. In 1970 control measures were introduced using N. tritylmorpholine as a molluscicide and niridazole as a drug against the adult parasites in the human population. The control measures were continued for four years and there was a year of post-control surveillance. During this follow-up period it was found that while transmission through *B. rohlfsi* had been virtually eliminated, transmission through *B. camerunensis* had risen to three times the pre-control level. Throughout the control period *B. camerunensis* had proved to be far less susceptible to N. tritylmorpholine, even when the dosage was increased well beyond the usual level, than had *B. rohlfsi*, thus selective elimination by more frequent treatments of the usual host for *S. haematobium* would have exerted a pressure on the parasite population in favour of those larvae able to develop in *B. camerunensis*. Wright *et al.* (1972) summarised evidence to suggest that at some time hybridisation between *S. haematobium* and *S. intercalatum* had occurred at Barombi Kotto and it is likely that the selection pressure of the molluscicide treatment favoured the parasites carrying *S. intercalatum* genes, for these would have been the ones most infective for *B. camerunensis*. At the same time the effect of this selection would have been enhanced by the drug treatment used against the adult worms for *S. intercalatum* has been shown to be more resistant than *S. haematobium* to niridazole (Brumpt *et al.*, 1968). Thus the dual control measures used at this focus appear to have selected from the existing hybrid population a strain of parasite which is unlikely to be amenable to control by the methods which are currently employed widely. It may well be that this isolated example provides a warning as to the possible outcome of more extensive schemes elsewhere.

ACKNOWLEDGEMENTS

We are grateful to Mrs. N. Dias, Miss J.R.L. Lines, Mr. G.C. Ross and Mr. R.J. Knowles for their assistance with various aspects of the experimental work described in this paper.

REFERENCES

ARMSTRONG, J.C. (1965). Mating behaviour and development of schistosomes in the mouse. *Journal of Parasitology* **51**, 605-616.

BECQUET, R. (1967). Contribution à l'étude de la bilharziose à *Schistosoma intercalatum*. *Annales de la Societé Belgique de Médécine Tropicale* **47**, 35-60.

BORAY, J.C. (1966). Studies on the relative susceptibility of some lymnaeids to infection with *Fasciola hepatica* and *F. gigantica* and on the adaptation of *Fasciola* spp. *Annals of Tropical Medicine and Parasitology* **60**, 114-124.

BROWN, D.S. and WRIGHT, C.A. (1974). *Bulinus truncatus* as a potential intermediate host for *Schistosoma haematobium* on the Kano plain, Kenya. *Transactions of the Royal Society of Tropical Medicine and Hygiene* **68**, 341-342.

BRUMPT, L.C., DEGREMONT, A., BARBIER, M., CONEMBARAS, A. and LAVARDE, V. (1968). Le niridazole dans le traitement des quatres bilharzioses a *S. haematobium*, *S. mansoni*, *S. japonicum* et *S. intercalatum Presse méd.* **76**, 797-804.

COLES, G.C. (1970). A comparison of some isoenzymes of *Schistosoma mansoni* and *Schistosoma haematobium*. *Comparative Biochemistry and Physiology* **33**, 549-558.

COLES, G.C. (1971a). Variations in malate dehydrogenase isoenzymes of *Schistosoma mansoni*. *Comparative Biochemistry and Physiology* **38B**, 35-42.

COLES, G.C. (1971b). Alteration of *Schistosoma mansoni* malate dehydrogenase isoenzymes on passage in the laboratory. *Comparative Biochemistry and Physiology* **40B**, 1079-1083.

DAVIS, G.M. (1968). A systematic study on *Oncomelania hupensis chiui* (Gastropoda: Hydrobiidae). *Malacologia* **7**, 17-70.

DUKE, B.O.L. and MOORE, P.J. (in prep. a) Control of *Schistosoma haematobium* at the Barombi lake foci in Cameroon. II. The attack on the snail hosts, using N-tritylmorpholine, and its effect on transmission from snail to man.

DUKE, B.O.L. and MOORE, P.J. (in prep. b). Control of *Schistosoma haematobium* at the Barombi lake foci in Cameroon, IV. The attack on the parasite in man, using niridazole, and its effect on transmission from man to snail.

FAN, P.C., PAO, K.Y. and LEE, M.C. (1974). Susceptibility of *Biomphalaria glabrata* and *Oncomelania hupensis chiui* to hybrid miracidia of schistosomes. *Proceedings of the 3rd International Congress of Parasitology* **2**, 808-809.

FRANDSEN, F. (1975). Host-parasite relationship of *Bulinus forskalii* (Ehrenberg) and *Schistosoma intercalatum* Fisher 1934, from Cameroun. *Journal of Helminthology* **49**, 73-84.

HARDING, J.P. (1949). The use of probability paper for the graphical analysis of polymodal frequency distributions. *Journal of the Marine Biological Association of the United Kingdom* **28**, 141-153.

HOWALDT, H.G. and ARMSTRONG, F.I. (1969). Susceptibilities of *Bulinus* (*Physopsis*) *africanus* and *B. truncatus* to four schistosome strains. *Transactions of the Royal Society of Tropical Medicine and Hygiene* **63**, 149-150.

HOWALDT, H.G. and PITCHFORD, R.J. (1963). Susceptibility of *Australorbis glabratus* & *Biomphalaria pfeifferi* to *Schistosoma rodhaini*. *Transactions of the Royal Society of Tropical Medicine and Hygiene* **57**, 313.

LE ROUX, P.L. (1954a). Hybridisation of *Schistosoma mansoni* and *Schistosoma rodhaini*. *Transactions of the Royal Society of Tropical Medicine and Hygiene* **48**, 3-4.

LE ROUX, P.L. (1954b). *Schistosoma* spp. recovered experimentally, through snails and mice and hamsters from a human subject of urinary schistosomiasis. *Transactions of the Royal Society of Tropical Medicine and Hygiene* **48**, 281.

MAO, S.P. (1962). Important achievements in the control of Bilharziasis in New China. *In Bilharziasis*. G.E.W. Wolstenholme and M. O'Connor (eds.) pp. 198-206. London: J. and A. Churchill.

PAPERNA, I. (1968). Susceptibility of *Bulinus globosus* and *Bulinus truncatus rohlfsi* from different localities in Ghana to different local strains of *Schistosoma haematobium*. *Annals of Tropical Medicine and Parasitology* **62**, 13-26.

PITCHFORD, R.J. (1959). Cattle schistosomiasis in man in the Eastern Transvaal. *Transactions of the Royal Society of Tropical Medicine and Hygiene* **53**, 285-290.

PITCHFORD, R.J. (1961). Observations on a possible hybrid between the two schistosomes *S. haematobium* and *S. mattheei*. *Transactions of the Royal Society of Tropical Medicine and Hygiene* **55**, 44-51.

PITCHFORD, R.J. (1965). Differences in the egg morphology and certain biological characteristics of some African & Middle eastern schistosomes, genus *Schistosoma*, with terminal-spined eggs. *Bulletin of the World Health Organization* **32**, 105-120.

ROSS, G.C. (in press). Isoenzymes in *Schistosoma* spp: LDH, MDH and acid phosphatases separated by isoelectric focusing in polyacrylamide gel. *Comparative Biochemistry and Physiology B.*

SAOUD, M.F. (1965). Changes in Egyptian *Schistosoma mansoni* by passage in *Biomphalaria glabrata* for 15 years. *Journal of Helminthology* **39**, 363-76.

SAOUD, M.F.A. (1966). Susceptibility of some planorbid snails to infection with *Schistosoma rodhaini* from Kenya. *Journal of Helminthology* **40**, 379-384.

SEVERINGHAUS, A.E. (1928). Sex studies on *Schistosoma japonicum*. *Quarterly Journal of Microscopical Science* **71**, 653-707.

SHORT, R.B. (1948). Intergeneric crosses among schistosomes. (Trematoda: Schistosomatidae). *Journal of Parasitology* **34**, (suppl.) 30.

SHORT, R.B. (1952a). Sex studies on *Schistosomatium douthitti* (Cort, 1914) Price, 1931 (Trematoda: Schistosomatidae). *American Midland Naturalist* **47**, 1-54.

SHORT, R.B. (1952b). Uniparental miracidia of *Schistosomatium douthitti* and their progeny (Trematoda: Schistosomatidae). *American Midland Naturalist* **48**, 55-68.

SHORT, R.B. (1957). Chromosomes and sex in *Schistosomatium douthitti*. *Journal of Heredity* **48**, 2-6.

SHORT, R.B. and MENZEL, M.Y. (1959). Chromosomes in parthenogenetic miracidia and embryonic cercariae of *Schistosomatium douthitti*. *Experimental Parasitology* **8**, 249-264.

SHORT, R.B. and MENZEL, M.Y. (1960). Chromosomes of nine species of Schistosomes. *Journal of Parasitology* **46**, 273-287.

SOUTHGATE, V.R. and KNOWLES, R.J. (1975). Observations on *Schistosoma bovis* Sonsino, 1876. *Journal of Natural History* **9**, 273-314.

SOUTHGATE, V.R. and KNOWLES, R.J. (1975). The intermediate hosts of *Schistosoma bovis* in Western Kenya. *Transactions of the Royal Society of Tropical Medicine and Hygiene* **69**, 356-357.

SOUTHGATE, V.R., van WIJK, H.B. and WRIGHT, C.A. (in press). Schistosomiasis at Loum, Cameroun; *Schistosoma haematobium, S. intercalatum* and their natural hybrid. *Zeitschrift für Parasitenkunde.*

TAYLOR, M.G. (1970). Hybridisation experiments on five species of African schistosomes. *Journal of Helminthology* **44**, 253-314.

TAYLOR, M.G. (1971). Comparative parasitology studies on African schistosomes and their hybrids in experimental infections. *Comptes-rendus 1er Multicolloque Européen de Parasitologie (Rennes, 1971)* 405-407.

TAYLOR, M.G. (1973). A comparison of the susceptibility to niridazole of *Schistosoma mansoni* and *S. intercalatum* in mice. *Transactions of the Royal Society of Tropical Medicine and Hygiene* **67**, 245-249.

TAYLOR, M.G., AMIN, M.B.A. and NELSON, G.S. (1969). "Parthenogenesis" in *Schistosoma mattheei. Journal of Helminthology* **43**, 197-206.

TAYLOR, M.G. and ANDREWS, B.J. (1973). Comparison of the infectivity and pathogenicity of six species of African schistosomes and their hybrids. 1. Mice and hamsters. *Journal of Helminthology* **47**, 439-453.

TAYLOR, M.G., NELSON, G.S., SMITH, M. and ANDREWS, B.J. (1973). Comparison of the infectivity and pathogenicity of six species of African schistosomes and their hybrids. 2. Baboons. *Journal of Helminthology* **47**, 455-485.

VOGEL, H. (1941). Uber den Einfluss des Geschlechts—partners auf Wachstum und Entwicklung bei *Bilharzia mansoni* und Kreuzpaarungen zivischen verschiedenen *Bilharzia*-Arten. *Zentralblatt für Bakteriologie und Parasitenkunde.* Abth 1. Orig. **148**, 78-96.

VOGEL, H. (1942). Uber die Nachkommenschaft aus Kreuzparungen zivischen. *Bilharzia mansoni* und *B. japonica. Zentralblatt für Bakteriologie und Parasitenkunde.* Abth 1. Orig. **149**, 319-333.

WRIGHT, C.A. (1960). Relationships between trematodes and molluscs. *Annals of Tropical Medicine and Parasitology* **54**, 1-7.

WRIGHT, C.A. (1962). The significance of infra-specific taxonomy in bilharziasis. In *Bilharziasis.* G.E.W. Wolstenholme and M. O'Connor (eds.) pp. 103-126. London: J. and A. Churchill.

WRIGHT, C.A. (1970). The ecology of African schistosomiasis. *In Human Ecology in the Tropics.* J.P. Garlick and R.W.J. Keay (eds). pp. 67-80. London: Pergamon Press.

WRIGHT, C.A. (1974). Snail susceptibility or trematode infectivity? *Journal of Natural History* **8**, 545-548.

WRIGHT, C.A. and BENNETT, M.S. (1967a). Studies on *Schistosoma haematobium* in the laboratory I. A strain from Durban, Natal, South Africa. *Transactions of the Royal Society of Tropical Medicine and Hygiene* **61**, 221-227.

WRIGHT, C.A. and BENNETT, M.S. (1967b). Studies on *Schistosoma haematobium* in the laboratory. II. A strain from South Arabia. *Transactions of the Royal Society of Tropical Medicine and Hygiene* **61**, 228-233.

WRIGHT, C.A. and KNOWLES, R.J. (1972). Studies on *Schistosoma haematobium* in the laboratory. III. Strains from Iran, Mauritius and Ghana. *Transactions of the Royal Society of Tropical Medicine and Hygiene* **66**, 108-118.

WRIGHT, C.A., SOUTHGATE, V.R. and KNOWLES, R.J. (1972). What is *Schistosoma intercalatum* Fisher, 1934? *Transactions of the Royal Society of Tropical Medicine and Hygiene* **66**, 28-64.

WRIGHT, C.A., SOUTHGATE, V.R., VAN WIJK, H.B. and MOORE, P.J. (1974). Hybrids between *Schistosoma haematobium* and *S. intercalatum* in Cameroon. *Transactions of the Royal Society of Tropical Medicine and Hygiene* **68**, 413-414.

THE ECOLOGICAL GENETICS OF HOST-PARASITE RELATIONSHIPS

BRYAN CLARKE

Department of Genetics, University Park,
Nottingham NG7 2RD

INTRODUCTION

Population geneticists have recently been concerned to explain the great extent of intra-specific genetic variation in proteins. Studies by Harris (1966) on man, and by Lewontin and Hubby (1966) on *Drosophila*, suggested that about 30 per cent of the structural genes for soluble enzymes are genetically polymorphic. Although it is now clear that various classes of enzymes (and of other proteins) differ in their propensities to polymorphism, work on a wide range of organisms has confirmed that the majority of outbreeding species are very variable indeed at the enzyme level. In some cases the observed proportion of polymorphic enzyme loci has been as high as 70 per cent (for reviews see Selander and Johnson, 1973; Selander and Kaufman, 1973). In seeking an explanation for this extraordinary degree of variability, there have been two major schools of thought. The first (the "neutralist" school) has argued that the majority of genetic variants are of little or no consequence to the survival and reproduction of the individuals manifesting them, and that the polymorphisms are maintained by a combination of mutation and random genetic drift (see, for example, Kimura and Ohta, 1971; Nei, 1975). The second school (the "selectionist" school) has argued that the majority of polymorphisms are actively maintained by natural selection. Their argument implies not only that the genetic variants significantly affect survival and reproduction, but also that selective "feedback mechanisms" act to restore genetic equilibrium when it is disturbed (Richmond, 1970; Clarke, 1970, 1975a).

The dispute between "neutralists" and "selectionists" has been long and hard, but it seems to be approaching a resolution. There is now increasing evidence that the amino-acid substitutions involved in protein polymorphisms significantly alter the biochemical properties of the proteins (Harris, 1971) and that the differences are subject to natural selection (Clarke, 1975a). However, a major difficulty has been to find the selective agents responsible for maintaining these polymorphisms.

In the present essay I shall argue that genetic interactions between parasites and their hosts have played an important, perhaps even a dominant,

87

part in maintaining protein polymorphisms. This possibility was first suggested in a prescient but neglected paper by the late J.B.S. Haldane (1949). Since that time we have learned a great deal more about the nature of host-parasite interactions, and the case has become very much stronger.

In presenting this case, I shall first state the arguments in the form of a series of hypotheses, and briefly review the evidence in their favour. Then I shall reformulate the hypotheses in terms of some very simple mathematical models, and examine their consequences for evolutionary theory.

THE HYPOTHESES

HYPOTHESIS 1

We know that there are mutual phenotypic adjustments between hosts and their parasites. If a host is initially uniform in its genetic composition, and if

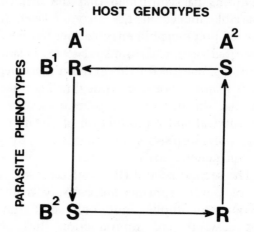

Fig. 1. A simple model of host-parasite interaction (corresponding to hypothesis 1; see text). The host is assumed to be haploid, and to manifest one of two possible alleles (A^1 and A^2). Hosts with A^1 are relatively resistant (R) to parasites of type B^1, but relatively susceptible (S) to parasites of type B^2. Hosts with A^2 are relatively resistant to B^2, but relatively susceptible to B^1. Apart from their effects on resistance and susceptibility, the genotypes are assumed to be equal in selective value. The arrows show the directions in which the frequencies of genes and phenotypes are expected to move. In the host, gene frequencies will move towards a preponderance of resistant genotypes. In the parasite, the phenotype frequencies will move towards a preponderance of forms to which the host is susceptible. The fact that the arrows form a closed circuit indicates that the system is potentially capable of maintaining polymorphisms in both species. Note that the phenotypes of the parasite may represent genotypes or environmentally-determined variants.

a parasite is finely adapted to the conditions of life in the host, then even a small biochemical change in the host might confer some degree of resistance against the parasite. Consequently, as Haldane pointed out, a host with a rare biochemical phenotype can gain a selective advantage. It follows, if the phenotype is genetically determined, that the corresponding genotype will increase in frequency. As its frequency increases, the advantage will decline because natural selection will favour variant parasites that can more effectively attack the new type of host. The appropriate phenotypes in the parasite will then begin to spread. Their subsequent behaviour will depend upon their relative success in attacking the original type of host. If they are able equally to infect both host genotypes, and are equally fit in other respects, they may spread to fixation. Then, in effect, the original state will be restored. If, however, an increased success in attacking the new host genotype carries with it a reduced ability to attack the old, a "feedback loop" may be established, in which polymorphisms are actively maintained in both host and parasite (see Fig. 1).

In diploid hosts the likelihood of polymorphism will be increased if the alleles for resistance are co-dominant, so that heterozygous hosts can resist two types of parasites. In diploid parasites, if the ability to attack particular types of host is genetically determined, the likelihood of polymorphism in both parasites and hosts will be increased when the genes concerned are co-dominant, so that heterozygous parasites can infect two homozygous types of hosts.

HYPOTHESIS 2

Even if the parasite is unable genetically or phenotypically to respond to the resistant host (i.e. if the host genotype confers a "general", rather than a "specific", resistance) a polymorphism can still be maintained in the host. This requires that the numbers of parasites are to some extent determined by the availability of susceptible hosts. When a gene for general resistance is rare, there will be many parasites, and relatively strong selection in favour of resistant genotypes. When the gene is common, there will be fewer parasites, and weaker selection in favour of resistant genotypes. The selective value of a resistant genotype will therefore be negatively related to its frequency. If the resistance gene has pleiotropic effects that are disadvantageous, there will be some frequency at which the advantageous and disadvantageous effects exactly cancel each other. This will be a stable equilibrium point (or there will be a stable limit cycle, see below), and polymorphism will be maintained.

Of course, if the gene for general resistance is dominant, but disadvantageous in the homozygous condition, polymorphism will be maintained by the heterozygous advantage, and it will be relatively insensitive to the number of parasites.

HYPOTHESIS 3

There is another way in which a gene for general resistance can be kept in the polymorphic state. If the parasite is patchy in its distribution, so that some populations of the host are attacked but others are not, the resistance gene may only be favoured in some places. If the gene has disadvantageous pleiotropic effects, selection will act against it where the parasite is absent. However, gene-flow between the two types of host population may ensure that both alleles are maintained in both types of population.

Assumptions underlying the hypotheses

The hypotheses given above depend upon the following assumptions:
1. That there is genetic variation in the ability of hosts to resist parasites.
2. That there is phenotypic variation in the ability of parasites to attack hosts. (Hypothesis 1).
3. That there are specific relations between these two types of variation (particularly, that an increased ability on the part of the host to resist one type of parasite reduces its ability to resist another). (Hypothesis 1).
4. That the numbers of parasites depend on the numbers of susceptible hosts. (Hypothesis 2).
5. That the variation in the host can show itself as protein polymorphism.
6. That the mortality (or reduced fertility) caused by parasites is great enough for it to be a major evolutionary force.
7. That the conditions for polymorphism following from host-parasite interactions are sufficiently robust that these interactions are likely to be common factors in maintaining genetic variability.

THE EVIDENCE

The evidence in favour of the first six assumptions will briefly be reviewed in this section. The evidence in favour of the seventh will be examined in the following section.

1. GENETIC VARIATION IN THE
ABILITY OF HOSTS TO RESIST
PARASITES

There can be no doubt that hosts generally vary in their ability to resist parasites, and that much of this variation in inherited. Bacteria rapidly develop genetic resistance to bacteriophages (see, for example, Horne, 1970). The widespread genetic variation in the resistance of plants to insects, fungi and bacteria has recently been reviewed by Day (1974). For animals the evidence is more diffuse but still compelling. We know of inherited variation in the resistance of houseflies to parasitic wasps (Olson and Pimentel, 1974), snails to schistosomes (Richards, this volume), rabbits to myxoma virus (Fenner, 1965) and men to malaria (Motulsky, 1975; Miller *et al.*, 1975). The importance of the histocompatibility polymorphisms to disease resistance among mice and men is reviewed by Bodmer (1972) and Vogel (1975). Selection for disease resistance among domestic animals has been an important part of our agricultural development. The list of possible examples is very long.

2. PHENOTYPIC VARIATION IN THE ABILITY OF PARASITES TO ATTACK HOSTS

As we shall see, for maintaining polymorphism among hosts it is not necessary that the variation among parasites should be genetic. The variant parasites may be different genotypes, but equally they may be different environmentally-determined varieties. Nonetheless, there is good evidence that genetic variation does occur. It is known in viruses, bacteria, fungi, trematodes and insects (for examples, see Fenner, 1965; Day, 1974; Richards, this volume). Examples of environmentally-determined phenotypic variations are given below.

3. RELATIONSHIPS BETWEEN THE GENOTYPES OF HOSTS AND THE PHENOTYPES OF THEIR PARASITES

That there can be precise relations between the genotypes of a host and the phenotypes of its parasite was first made clear by Flor (1956) in his studies on the interaction between flax (*Linum usitatissimum*) and flax rust (*Melampsora lini*). He showed that during their evolution the host and parasite have developed complementary genetic arrangements and that "for each gene conditioning rust reaction in the host, there is a specific gene conditioning pathogenicity in the parasite". Following Flor, gene-for-gene relationships between parasite and host have been found in seven plant-fungus systems (Day, 1974), and also in the relations between wheat (*Triticum*) and an *insect* parasite, *Mayetiola destructor* (Hatchett and Gallun, 1970). The last example is important because it shows that the phenomenon is not restricted to plants. Mode (1958) and Person (1959; 1966) have argued that this type of system can maintain polymorphisms in both interacting species.

It has been suggested that gene-for-gene relationships may also occur between vertebrate hosts and their parasites (Damian, 1964; see also Rowley and Jenkin, 1962; Dineen, 1963). It is argued that a parasite in an immunologically competent host could protect itself by reducing the antigenic disparity between itself and the host (i.e. by "mimicking" the host's antigens). Since an organism cannot normally react against its own antigens, the parasite would then be protected from immunological attack. This would produce selection in favour of antigenically variant hosts that could damage the parasite.

There is now a wide, if inconsistent, literature on antigen sharing between host and parasite (reviewed by Damian, 1964). Many species of bacteria are known to cross-react immunologically with ABO blood group and HL-A histocompatibility antisera (Mittal *et al.*, 1973). There is evidence of antigens shared between parasitic nematodes and trematodes and their mammalian hosts (Damian, 1964). These antigens may persist when the parasites are removed from the species with which they cross-react, and are grown in a different host (Damian *et al.*, 1973).

Because there are often antigenic similarities between unrelated organisms that are *not* involved in common parasite-host relationships, and because there are cross-reactions between parasites of plants and the plants they inhabit (de Vay, *et al.*, 1972), there is some doubt whether mammalian parasites have acquired their cross-reacting antigens as a result of immunological selection, or whether they have done so because of some other form of selection, or indeed whether the phenomenon is fortuitous. In any of these cases, however, the presence of shared antigens could act to promote polymorphism in the host.

The same argument applies to situations in which the antigens on the surfaces of parasites are not genetic at all, but are acquired from their hosts. A rare antigenic type of host would gain a temporary advantage if its potential invaders carried antigens of the common type. The well-known tendency of many viruses to wrap themselves in the cell-membranes of their hosts should therefore promote antigenic polymorphism. The existence of antigenic polymorphisms that are known to be associated with differential resistance to various infectious diseases adds strength to these arguments (Bodmer, 1972; Vogel, 1975). The associations with viral infections are particularly clear.

Although specific relationships between the genotypes of vertebrate hosts and the phenotypes of their parasites have been most thoroughly discussed at the immunological level, it seems almost certain that they will occur at other levels as well. The elegant work of Fenner (1965) has shown a continuous mutual genetic adjustment between the rabbit and the myxoma virus, an adjustment that is unlikely to be entirely immunological. It also seems unlikely that *Plasmodium falciparum* has failed to adjust genetically to the changes in its environment brought about by the occurrence of abnormal haemoglobin, deficient glucose-6-phosphate dehydrogenases, or raised ATP levels, among its "resistant" hosts.

4. THE NUMBERS OF PARASITES DEPENDENT UPON THE NUMBERS OF SUSCEPTIBLE HOSTS

It is almost a tautology to say that the numbers of parasites must depend upon the numbers of susceptible hosts, yet some care is needed when we are discussing the coevolution of two individual species. For example, it seems unlikely that the numbers of *Plasmodium knowlesi*, a simian parasite, will be much affected by small differences in the susceptibilities of men. The numbers of relatively susceptible or resistant monkeys would be another matter. Thus if we are to appeal to a model that demands a relation between the gene frequencies of the host and the numbers of the parasite, we must apply it only to the (or a) major host species.

That such relations can exist is shown by the success of resistant varieties of crops in (temporarily) reducing the numbers of pests.

5. PROTEIN POLYMORPHISM AS AN EXPRESSION OF SEGREGATING GENES FOR RESISTANCE

It is known that segregating genes for resistance to parasites can show themselves as electrophoretically detectable protein polymorphisms. The variant haemoglobins S and C, and the "deficient" variant of glucose-6-phosphate dehydrogenase, which confer resistance to malaria, are obvious examples. The transferrin polymorphism in pigeons (Frelinger, 1972) seems to be another. The histocompatibility antigens, and many blood group antigens, are proteins, although detecting their variants by electrophoresis would be difficult because they are so closely bound to the cell membrane. However, two electrophoretically detectable serum proteins that are components of the complement system segregate with the major histocompatibility (H-2) locus in mice. Their products must be intimately concerned with the ability to react to parasites. Furthermore, it seems certain that the majority of "non-protein" antigenic polymorphisms reflect an underlying variation at the protein level. The ABO blood groups in man, for example, which apparently influence resistance to influenza A2 and to adenoviruses, and which are detected because of the antigenic properties of their carbohydrate chains, nevertheless represent genetic differences in glycosyl transferase enzymes. We do not yet know if these differences are detectable by electrophoresis, although it seems likely that they would be if suitable staining techniques were available.

Strobel (1973) has recently established the nature of resistance to eyespot disease (*Helminthosporium sacchari*) in sugarcane. The fungus produces a host-specific toxin that binds to the cell-membrane of susceptible plants. Membranes prepared from resistant plants do not bind the toxin. Proteins from the two types of membrane were isolated, and found to differ in four amino acid residues. The difference between the proteins is thus directly associated with resistance to eyespot disease.

6. THE MORTALITY CAUSED BY PARASITES

Although it is often claimed that an efficient parasite does not kill its host, one should more properly say that an efficient parasite does not kill *all* its hosts. Even in these terms the world is full of moderately inefficient parasites. The devastating effects of malaria, yellow fever, plague, potato blight and dutch elm disease testify to this fact. However, in order to exercise efficient natural selection a parasite only has to kill *some* of its hosts. A parasite that is benign in times of plenty may still be a burden in times of stress.

The vast array of complex arrangements that organisms have evolved as defences against parasites, from the possession of hairy leaves to the development of antibodies, shows the power of parasites in determining the pattern of evolution. They are undoubtedly a most potent agent of natural selection.

In man a single group of related diseases, the malarias, is apparently responsible for selection acting on at least three polymorphisms (haemoglobin, glucose-6-phosphate dehydrogenase and the Duffy blood groups; see Motulsky, 1975; Miller *et al.*, 1975) and probably on several more (including the genes regulating levels of ATP, and perhaps some of the HL-A alleles: see Motulsky, 1975; Piazza *et al.*, 1973). If each major class of human disease has generated a similar crop of variants, then disease-related polymorphism may constitute a major component of human biochemical diversity. The same logic applies to other organisms.

THE MODELS

The assumptions underlying our hypotheses are realistic. Hosts do indeed show genetic variation in their ability to resist parasites, and parasites show phenotypic variation in their ability to attack hosts. There is good evidence of specificity in the relations between the two types of variation. The numbers of parasites may often depend upon the numbers of susceptible hosts. The variation in the host can manifest itself as protein polymorphism, and the mortality caused by parasites is sufficient to account for the maintenance of a large number of such polymorphisms.

The hypotheses can now be framed in more rigorous forms, as very simple mathematical models. I shall consider two models, the first corresponding to hypotheses 1 (Figure 1) with specific resistance genes, the second corresponding to hypothesis 2 and supposing a general resistance gene with a dependence of the numbers of parasites on the numbers of susceptible hosts. I shall not provide a model of hypothesis 3, but the potential of that system for maintaining polymorphism is self-evident.

1. A MODEL OF SPECIFIC RESISTANCE
(HYPOTHESIS 1)

There have been two theoretical studies of specific resistance in which mathematical models have been constructed. Mode (1958) examined the properties of a rather special system representing the gene-for-gene relations between flax and flax rust. Assuming continuous generations he was able to show that under some conditions there can be stable polymorphisms in both parasite and host. Yu (1972) constructed several models that are more general, corresponding approximately to the one shown in Figure 1. He found that there were stable non-trivial equilibria (with polymorphism in both parasite and host) only when the parasites were diploid and when the fitness of the heterozygote for two "virulence" genes exceeded the mean fitness of the two homozygotes. The following model makes slightly different assumptions from Yu's, and comes to very different conclusions.

I assume that the host is haploid. This assumption is made not only because it greatly simplifies the mathematcis, but also because the conditions for polymorphism in haploids are generally more stringent than those for polymorphisms in diploids. If this model predicts balance, many diploid models will also do so.

The host is assumed to have two genotypes A^1 and A^2. Their frequencies are p and $1-p$ respectively. There are two types of parasites, B^1 and B^2, with frequencies r and $1-r$ respectively. A^1 hosts are relatively resistant to B^1 parasites and relatively susceptible to B^2. A^2 hosts are relatively resistant to B^2 and relatively susceptible to B^1. The numbers of hosts and parasites are assumed to remain constant from generation to generation. Encounters

BRYAN CLARKE

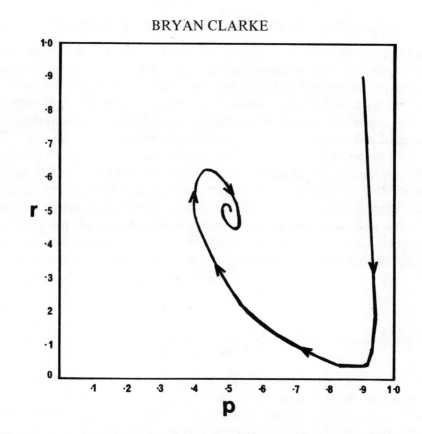

Fig. 2. A simulation of the model of specific resistance when s = 0.25 and t = 0.60. Note that the gene frequencies move to a stable equilibrium.

between particular types of hosts and parasites are supposed to occur in proportion to their frequencies. Thus the proportion of A^1-B^1 encounters will be pr, of A^1-B^2 encounters $p(1-r)$, and so on. 1 assume that when hosts meet parasites to which they are relatively resistant, a proportion s of the hosts is killed, and that the parasites emerging from them are now able to infect hosts of the same genotype (i.e. that a proportion of the parasites has changed from the kind that is relatively avirulent in this particular genotype of host to the kind that is relatively virulent; this could be the result either of selection for mutant parasites within the host, or because the parasites have been phenotypically changed by the host environment—for example by wrapping themselves in the host membrane). The remaining proportion ($1-s$) of hosts survives, and kills the parasites. I assume that when a host meets a parasite to which it is relatively susceptible, a proportion t ($t > s$) is killed, and that the parasites emerging from them are able to infect hosts of the same genotype (i.e. no relevant genetic or phenotypic change takes place).

The remaining proportion (*l-t*) of hosts survives and kills the parasites. In the next generations, the relative numbers of the different kinds of parasite are determined by, and proportional to, the numbers of their hosts that are killed.

Following these assumptions we find that in the next generation the new frequency of A^1 is

$$p' = \frac{p(1-t-r(s-t))}{1-s-(s-t)(2pr-p-r)}$$

and the new frequency of B^1 is

$$r' = \frac{(1-p)(s-r(s-t))}{s+(s-t)(2pr-p-r)}$$

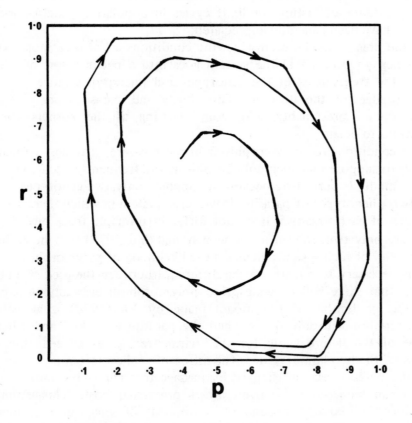

Fig. 3. A simulation of the model of specific resistance, when s = 0.10 and t = 0.75. Note that the gene frequencies converge on a stable limit cycle.

The recurrence relations allow us to investigate the properties of the system, using different values of s and t. Under some conditions the system moves to a single stable non-trivial equilibrium ($\hat{p} = 0.5$, $\hat{r} = 0.5$) at which both hosts and parasites are kept in the polymorphic state (Fig. 2). These conditions can be specified, but they need not concern us because *under all other conditions, except when $s = 0$ or $t = 1$, the system moves into a stable limit cycle which will also maintain joint polymorphisms in hosts and parasites* (Fig. 3).

The matter of limit cycles is important because it is a common practise in theoretical population genetics to locate points of equilibrium and to investigate their stability. If all internal equilibria are unstable, the system is often supposed to be incapable of maintaining polymorphism. Because stable limit cycles are potential consequences of many non-linear interacting systems, the supposition may often be incorrect. May (1972) has forcefully made this point in relation to ecological models, and Jayakar (1970) and Yu (1972) have observed cycles in some of their host-parasite systems. However, the importance of testing for limit cycles in population genetics does not seem to have been generally appreciated.

In the present model even when the conditions are at their most extreme (i.e. when $s = 0$ or $t = 1$) the system goes into a peculiar sort of cycle, in which the frequencies of the genotypes and phenotypes move round the outside edge of the diagram. Thus hosts and parasites are alternately polymorphic, presumably with some waiting at the corners for new mutations to occur.

The conditions for polymorphisms in the host are extremely robust, and lead us to suppose that such polymorphisms will frequently occur.

The model is unrealistic because it supposes only two genotypes of host, and two phenotypes of parasite. However, a system in which there are many varieties of each organism does not differ in principle from one in which there are only two. Indeed it has been argued (Yu, 1972) that increasing the complexity of such systems increases the likelihood of polymorphism.

It is necessary to remark on the difference between the prediction of my model, that there will be widespread polymorphism even among haploids, and the prediction of the model made by Yu (1972), that balanced polymorphism will only occur when the parasite is diploid and when the fitness of the heterozygote for the "virulence" genes exceeds the mean fitness of the two homozygotes. The difference follows from my assumption that the parasite can be changed by passage through a "resistant" host, so that it can then more effectively attack other such hosts. This assumption introduces a frequency-dependent component of selection that tends to balance the system. Since changes during passage through "resistant" hosts are well known, my assumption makes the model more realistic.

2. A MODEL OF GENERAL RESISTANCE
(HYPOTHESIS 2)

To my knowledge, no models of "general" resistance have been proposed. Jayakar (1970) has suggested a model for "general virulence" in which the pattern of resistance (R) and susceptibility (S) are of the form:

		Host genotypes	
		A^1	A^2
parasite	B^1	S	R
genotypes	B^2	S	S

He found that balanced polymorphisms are not maintained, but that a "neutral" (unbalanced) polymorphism in the host can arise when the virulent (B^2) parasite spreads to fixation before the "resistant" (A^2) host has done so. This, of course, requires that the response of the parasite is more rapid than that of the host. Jayakar assumed that the number of parasites and hosts were constant.

We can propose a very simple model of general resistance. Suppose there are two host genotypes, A^1 which is susceptible to all forms of the parasite and A^2 which is completely resistant to all forms, but which suffers a pleiotropic disadvantage that can be represented by a constant component of fitness (l-s). The frequencies of A^1 and A^2 are p and l-p respectively. Let us also suppose that the numbers of parasites infecting the next generation are linearly related to the numbers of susceptible hosts, and that the fraction of susceptible hosts infected is proportional to the numbers of parasites. These assumptions of linearity are not realistic, but err in the right direction, because when the numbers of parasites are small the number of infected hosts is likely to be disproportionately smaller.

We have:

genotype	A^1	A^2
frequency	p	l-p
selective value	l-kp	l-s

where s and k are constants ($k<1$, $s<1$). It is easy to show that there is a single non-trivial equilibrium when

$$\hat{p} = \frac{s}{k}$$

and that this equilibrium is stable.

When the "resistant" form is not totally resistant, we can write the selective values of A^1 and A^2 as *1-kp* and *(1-s)(1-kp(1-x))* respectively, where x is constant ($x<1$) and measures the degree of resistance. Once more we find a single, stable non-trivial equilibrium:

$$\hat{p} = \frac{s(1-k(1-x))}{kx}$$

These equilibria are stable for all values of *s, k* and *x* between 0 and 1. Thus the conditions for polymorphism are very robust, particularly when we remember that the model errs in reducing the balancing effects. We note that if the relations between numbers of susceptible genotypes, numbers of parasites, and selective values are non-linear, there is again the possibility of stable limit cycles.

CONCLUSIONS

We may conclude that interactions between parasites and hosts can give rise to balanced polymorphisms in the hosts under a very wide range of circumstances. The models corresponding to hypotheses 1 and 2 above are robust in their predictions of balance. No model for hypothesis 3 has been given, but its balancing capacity is self-evident.

Although the hypotheses have been treated separately, the natural interaction between parasites and hosts is almost certain to encompass all three. The likelihood of balanced polymorphism would then be further enhanced. Both theory and observation indicate that the selection exerted by parasites on their hosts is density-dependent as well as frequency-dependent. Some properties of frequency-dependent and density-dependent selection have already been explored (Clarke, 1972; 1975b) and we know that they are potentially capable of maintaining large numbers of polymorphisms without the conventional problems of genetic load.

The variants subject to natural selection by parasites will often be detected as amino acid substitutions in proteins. It therefore seems reasonable to conclude that interactions between parasites and their hosts have played an important, perhaps even a dominant, role in maintaining protein polymorphisms.

POSTSCRIPT

It is worth drawing attention to the fact that frequency-dependent selection will not only maintain diversity within species, but also promote divergence between them (Haldane, 1949; Clarke, 1962; Bulmer, 1974). If two closely-related species of hosts share one or more species of parasite, it will be advantageous for the hosts to diverge. Variants of either host that depart from the other will tend to be favoured by natural selection. This pressure may be a significant factor in the interspecific evolution of proteins. Nor need it be restricted to proteins. There is a real possibility that the very striking diversity in DNA composition (GC ratio) between groups of bacteria may have evolved as a way of preventing infection by foreign DNA. The same may be true of the differences in the composition of highly-repeated DNA sequences between species of higher animals (Pardue, 1975). It has been suggested that one of the functions of these sequences is to guard against attack by viruses (Hsu, 1975). The forces that promote diversity between species will also tend to balance their relative numbers.

ACKNOWLEDGEMENTS

I am very grateful to Professor D.J. Bradley, Dr. T.H. Day, Dr. R.G. Lloyd and Dr. D.T. Parkin for critically reading the manuscript, and to the Science Research Council for financial support.

LITERATURE CITED

BODMER, W.F. (1972). Evolutionary significance of the HL-A system. *Nature*, **237**, 139-145.

BULMER, M.G. (1974). Density-dependent selection and character displacement. *American Naturalist*. **108**, 45-58.

CLARKE, B. (1962). Balanced polymorphism and the diversity of sympatric species. In: *Taxonomy and Geography* D. Nichols, ed. Systematics Association, Oxford.

CLARKE, B. (1970). The Darwinian evolution of proteins. *Science* **168**, 1009-1011.

CLARKE, B. (1972). Density-dependent selection. *American Naturalist* **106**, 1-13.

CLARKE, B. (1975a). The contribution of ecological genetics to evolutionary theory: detecting the direct effects of natural selection on particular polymorphic loci. *Genetics Suppl.* **79**, 101-113.

CLARKE, B. (1975b). Frequency-dependent and density-dependent selection. In: *The Role of Natural Selection in Human Evolution* F.M. Salzano, ed., North-Holland, Amsterdam.

DAY, P.R. (1974). *Genetics of host-parasite interaction.* W.H. Freeman, San Francisco.

DAMIAN, R.T. (1964). Molecular mimicry: antigen sharing by parasite and host and its consequences. *American Naturalist* **98**, 129-149.

DAMIAN, R.T. GREENE, N.D. and HUBBARD, W.J. (1973). Occurrence of mouse a_2-macroglobulin antigenic determinants on *Schistosoma mansoni* adults, with evidence of their nature. *Journal of Parasitology* **59**, 64-73.

DE VAY, J.E. CHARADATTAN, R., WIMALAJEEWA, D.L.S. (1972). Common antigenic determinants as a possible regulator of host-pathogen compatability. *American Naturalist* **106**, 185-194.

DINEEN, J.K. (1963). Immunological aspects of parasitism. *Nature* **197**, 268-269.

FENNER, F. (1965). Myxoma virus and *Oryctolagus cuniculus*: two colonizing species. In: *Genetics of Colonising Species* H.G. Baker and G.L. Stebbins, eds., Academic Press, New York.

FLOR, H.H. (1956). The complementary genetic systems in flax and flax rust. *Advances in Genetics* **8**, 29-54.

FRELINGER, J.A. (1972). The maintenance of transferrin polymorphism in pigeons. *Proceedings of the National Academy of Sciences, Washington* **69**, 326-329.

HALDANE, J.B.S. (1949). Disease and evolution. *La Ricerca Scientifica Suppl.* **19**, 68-76.

HARRIS, H. (1966). Enzyme polymorphisms in man. *Proceedings of the Royal Society of London Series B* **164**, 298-310.

HARRIS, H. (1971). Protein polymorphism in man. *Canadian Journal of Genetical Cytology* **13**, 381-396.

HATCHETT, J.H. and GALLUN, R.L. (1970). Genetics of the ability of the Hessian fly, *Mayetiola destructor*, to survive on wheats having different genes for resistances. *Annals of the Entomological Society of America* **63**, 185-194.

HORNE, M.T. (1970). Coevolution of *Escherichia coli* and bacteriophages in chemostat culture. *Science* **168**, 992-993.

HSU, T.C. (1975). A possible function of constitutive heterochromatin: the bodyguard hypothesis. *Genetics Supplement* **79**, 137-150.

JAYAKAR, S.D. (1970). A mathematical model of gene frequencies in a parasite and its host. *Theoretical Population Biology* **1**, 140-164.

KIMURA, M. and OHTA, T. (1971). *Theoretical Aspects of Population Genetics.* Princeton University Press, Princeton, N.J.

LEWONTIN, R.C. and HUBBY, J.L. (1966). A molecular approach to genic heterozygosity in natural populations. II. Amount of variation and degree of heterozygosity in natural populations of *Drosophila pseudoobscura*. *Genetics* **54**, 595-609.

MAY, R.M. (1972). Limit cycles in predator-prey communities. *Science* **177**, 900-902.

MILLER, L.H. MASON, S.J. DVORAK, J.A. McGINNISS, M.H. and ROTHMAN, I.K. (1975). Erythrocyte receptors for (*Plasmodium knowlesii*) malaria: Duffy blood group determinants. *Science* **189**, 561-563.

MITTAL, K.K. TERASAKI, P.I. SPRINGER, G.F. DESAI, P.R. McINTIRE, F.C. and HIRATA, A.A. (1973). Inhibition of anti-HL-A alloantisera by glycoproteins, polysaccharides, and lipopolysaccharides from diverse sources. *Transplantation Proceedings* **5**, 499-506.

MODE, C.J. (1958). A mathematical model for the coevolution of obligate parasites and their hosts. *Evolution, Lancaster, Pa.* **12**, 138-165.

MOTULSKY, A.G. (1975). Glucose-6-phosphate dehydrogenase and abnormal hemoglobin polymorphisms—evidence regarding malarial selection. In: *The Role of Natural Selection in Human Evolution* F.M. Salzano, ed., North-Holland, Amsterdam.

NEI, M. (1975). *Molecular Populations Genetics and Evolution*, North-Holland, Amsterdam.

OLSON, D.C. and PIMENTEL, D. (1974). Evolution of resistance in a host population to an attacking parasite. *Environmental Entomology* **3**, 621-624.

PARDUE, M.L. (1975). Repeated DNA sequences in the chromosomes of higher organisms. *Genetics Supplement* **79**, 159-170.

PERSON, C. (1959). Gene-for-gene relationships in host:parasite systems. *Canadian Journal of Botany* **37**, 1101-1130.

PERSON, C. (1966). Genetic polymorphism in parasitic systems. *Nature* **212**, 266-267.

PIAZZA, A. BELVEDERE, M.C. BERNOCO, D. CONIGHI, C. CONTU, L. CURTONI, E.S. MATTIUZI, P.L. MAYR, W. RICHIARDI, P. SCUDELLER, G. and CEPELLINI, R. (1973). HL-A variation in four Sardinian villages under differential selective pressure by malaria. In: *Histocompatibility Testing 1972*, J. Dausset and J. Colombani, eds., Munksgaard, Copenhagen.

RICHMOND, R.C. (1970). Non-Darwinian evolution: a critique. *Nature* **225**, 1025-1028.

ROWLEY, D. and JENKIN, C.R. (1962). Antigenic cross-reaction between host and parasite as a possible cause of pathogenicity. *Nature* **193**, 151-154.

SELANDER, R.K. and JOHNSON, W.E. (1973). Genetic variation among vertebrate species. *Annual Review of Ecological Systematics* **4**, 75-91.

SELANDER, R.K. and KAUFMAN, D.W. (1973). Genic variability and strategies of adaptation in animals. *Proceedings of the National Academy of Sciences, Washington* **70**, 1875-1877.

STROBEL, G.A. (1973). Biochemical basis of the resistance of sugarcane to eyespot disease. *Proceedings of the National Academy of Sciences, Washington* **70**, 1693-1696.

VOGEL, F. (1975). ABO blood groups, the HL-A system and diseases. In: *The Role of Natural Selection in Human Evolution* F.M. Salzano, ed., North-Holland, Amsterdam.

YU, P. (1972). Some host parasite genetic interaction models. *Theoretical Population Biology* **3**, 347-352.

AUTHOR INDEX

Numbers in heavy type refer to the pages on which references are listed
at the end of each paper

Adak, T., 19, **20**
Alger, N.E., 36, **41**
Allen, S.L., 28, **41**
Amin, M.B.A., **86**
Andrews, B.J., 58, 74, **86**
Arcolea, G., 37, **41**
Armstrong, F.I., 68, **84**
Armstrong, J.C., 56, **84**
Aslamkhan, M., 10, 17, **21**
Astin, J.K., **42**

Barbier, M., **84**
Barbosa, F.S., 45, **53**
Barr, A.J., 10, 11, **20**, **24**
Barreto, A.C., 45, **53**
Bartholomew, R., **43**
Becquet, R., 66, **84**
Belkin, J.N., 1, **20**
Belvedere, M.C., **103**
Bennett, M.S., 77, **86**
Bernoco, D., **103**
Bieniok, R., **21**
Bishop, 27, 30, **41**
Bodmer, W.F., 91, 92, **101**
Bond, H.W., 30, **42**
Boray, J.C., 81, **84**
Branton, M., **41**
Briggs, N.T., 35, **41**
Brown, D.S., 82, **84**
Brown, I.N., 35, **41**
Brown, K.N., 35, **41**
Bruce-Chwatt, L.J., **43**
Brumpt, L.C., 83, **84**
Bulmer, M.G., 101, **101**

Canning, E.U., 33, 41, **43**
Carriescia, P.M., 37, **41**
Carter, R., 25, 28, 41, 43, **44**
Ceppellini, R., **103**
Ceppellini, R., 37, **41**
Charadattan, R., **102**

Chellapah, W.T., 14. **20**
Chwatt, L.J., Bruce-, *see*
  Bruce-Chwatt, L.J.
Clarke, B., 87, 100, 101,
  101
Coatney, G.R., 42, **43**
Coles, G.C., 77, 79, **84**
Colless, D.H., 7, **20**
Conembaras, A., **84**
Conighi, C., **103**
Contu, L., **103**
Correa, L.R., 45, **53**
Coulston, F., 27, **41**
Cousserans, J., 17, 20, **21**
Cox, F.E.G., 35, **42**
Cox, H.W., 35, **42**
Craig, G.B., 13, **23**
Cram, E.B., 45, **53**
Curtis, C.F., 17, 18, 19,
  20, **23**
Curtoni, E.S., **103**

Damian, R.T., 91, 92, **101**
Das, M., **22**
Davidson, G., 16, **20**
Davis, G.M., 79, **84**
Day, P.R., 91, **101**
De Vay, J.E., 92, **102**
Degremont, A., **84**
Demidowa, L.W., 27, **42**
Desai, P.R., **102**
Desowitz, R.S., 14, **20**
Diggens, S.M., 28, 30, **42**
Dineen, J.K., 92, **102**
Downs, W.G., 27, **42**
Duke, B.O.L., 83, **84**
Dvorak, J.A., **102**

Entner, N., **43**
Ewert, A., 14, **20**

Fan, P.C., 58, 72, 79, **84**
Fenner, F., 91, 92, **102**
Files, V.S., 45, **53**
Fletcher, A., 40, **42**
Flor, H.H., 91, **102**
Frandsen, F., 71, 80, **84**
Frelinger, J.A., 93, **102**

Gallun, R.L., 91, **102**
Garnham, P.C.C., 31, **42**
Gibson, I., 28, **41**
Gilford, B.N., 5, 6, **23**
Greenberg, J., 30, 31, 32,
  37, **42**; 31, **43**
Greenberg, J., 31, **43**
Greene, N.D., **101**
Grover, K.K. **22**
Guille, G., 17, 20, **21**

Haldane, J.B.S., 88, 101,
  102
Hall, P., **43**
Harant, J., **41**
Harding, J.P., 62, **84**
Hargreaves, B.J., 40, 43, **44**
Harris, H., 87, **102**
Hatchett, J.H., 91, **102**
Henrard, C., 13, **21**
Herman, R., **42**
Hills, L.A., **41**
Hirata, A.A., **102**
Hitchcock, J.C., 5, **21**
Horne, M.T., 91, **102**
Howaldt, H.G., 68, 84, **85**
Hsu, T.C., 101, **102**
Huang, Y.M., 1, **21**
Hubbard, W.J., **101**
Hubby, J.L., 87, **102**

Jacobs, R.L., 37, **42**
Jayakar, 98, 99, **102**

Jenkin, C.R., 92, **103**
Johnson, W.E., 87, **103**
Jost, E., 17, **21**

Kalra, N.L., 15, **21**
Kaufman, D.W., 87, **103**
Kennedy, R. Killick-, *see*
    Killick-Kennedy, R.
Khalil, G.M., 14, **23**
Killick-Kendrick, R., 25,
    28, 40, **42**
Kimura, M., 87, **102**
Knowles, R.J., 55, 57, 59,
    60, 66, 68, 69, 71, 72,
    74, 77, 81, 82, **85**, **86**
Krishnamurthy, B.S., 10,
    18, **21**, **23**
Kuntz, R.E., 45, **53**

LaChance, L.E., 16, **22**
Lavarde, V., **84**
Laven, H., 9, 10, 16, 17,
    19, **21**
Lavoipierre, M.M.J., 14, **22**
Le Roux, P.L., 57, 59, 60,
    68, 72, **85**
Lee, M.C., **84**
Lewontin, R.C., 87, **102**
Luzzatto, L., 37, **42**

McClelland, G.A.H., 11, 14,
    21, **22**
McConnachie, E.W., 30, **41**
McDonald, P.T., 17, **22**
Macdonald, W.W., 13, 14,
    21, **22**
McGinniss, M.H., **102**
McGreevy, P.B., 14, **22**
McGregor, I.A., 28, **41**
McGregor, I.M., **43**
McIntire, F.C., **102**
Maegraith, B., 40, **42**
Mammen, M.L., 14, **22**
Manwell, R.D., 27, **41**
Mao, S.P., 79, **85**
Marks, E.N., 1, **22**
Mason, S.J., **102**
Mattiuzi, P.L., **103**
May, R.M., 98, **102**
Mayr, W., **103**
Menzel, M.Y., 48, 54; 56,
    85
Merritt, J.W., 46, **54**
Meyer, E., **21**
Miller, L.H., 91, 94, **102**

Mittal, K.K., 92, **102**
Mode, C.J., 91, 95, **102**
Moore, P.J. 83, **84**, **86**
Morgan, S., 30, 34, **42**, **43**
Most, H.M., 37, **42**, **43**
Motulsky, 91, 94, **102**

Nadel, E.M., **42**
National Institute of Com-
    municable Diseases,
    14, **22**
Nei, M., 87, **102**
Nelson, G.S., **86**
Newton, W.L., 52, **53**
Nussenzweig, R.S., **42**, **43**

Obiamiwe, B.A., 14, **22**
Oemijati, S., 14, **22**
Ogunba, E.O., 14, **22**
Ohmann, J., 17, **21**
Ohta, T., 87, **102**
Olson, D.C., 91, **102**
Ott, K.J., 37, **42**
Oxbrow, A.I., 31, 35, 36,
    37, **42**, **43**

Pal, R., 16, **22**
Pao, K.Y., **84**
Paperua, I., 82, **85**
Paraense, W.L., 45, **53**
Pardue, M.L., 101, **103**
Partono, F., 14, **22**
Perry, W.J., 9, **22**
Person, C., 91, **103**
Peters, W., 29, 37, **42**
Piazza, A., 94, **103**
Pimental, D., 91, **102**
Pitchford, R.J., 57, 60, 63,
    68, **85**

Raghavan, N.G.S., 14, **22**
Rai, K.S., 17, **22**, **23**
Ramachandran, C.P., 13,
    14, **22**, **23**
Rao, T.R., 16, **23**
Richards, C.S., 45, 46, 48,
    53, **54**
Richiardi, P., **103**
Richmond, R.C., 87, **103**
Rodriguez, P.H., 13, **23**
Ross, G.C., 77, 79, **85**
Rothman, I.K., **102**
Rowley, D., 92, **103**
Rozeboom, L.E., 5, 6, 15,
    21, **23**

Salaman, M.H., 37, **43**
Sanderson, A., **43**
Saoud, M.F., 81, **85**
Saoud, M.F.A., 68, **85**
Schacher, J.F., 14, **23**
Schoenfeld, C., 34, 35, **43**
Scudeller, G., **103**
Selander, R.K., 87, **103**
Severinghaus, A.E., 56, **85**
Sheppard, P.M., 13, **22**
Short, R.B., 48, **53**; 56, 58,
    85
Silverman, P.H., **41**
Sinden, R.E., 33, **41**, **43**
Singh, K.R.P., 14, **23**
Singh, N.N., 14, **22**
Smith, M., **86**
Smith-White, S., 7, 9, 10,
    11, **23**
Southgate, V.R., 55, 57,
    59, 60, 66, 68, 69, 71,
    72, 74, 77, 79, 81, 82,
    85, **86**
Springer, G.F., **102**
Stauber, L.A., **42**
Strobel, G.A., 94, **103**
Subbarao, 10, **23**
Suguna, S.G., 17, **22**

Tait, A., 28, **43**
Taylor, M.G., 58, 74, 75,
    86
Terasaki, P.I., **102**
Terwedow, H.A., 13, **23**
Tesfa-Yohannes, T.-M., 5,
    6, 15, **23**
Thomas, V., 14, **23**
Townson, H., 13, 16, **23**
Trembley, H.L., 26, 31, **42**,
    43

Upmanis, R.S., **43**, **44**
Uppal, D.K., 17, **23**

van Wijk, H.B. **86**
Vanderberg, J., **42**
Vay, J.E. de, *see* De Vay, J.E.
Vogel, H., 56, 58, **86**; 91,
    92, **103**
Voller, A., 35, **42**

Walker, P.J., 37, **43**
Walliker, D., 26, 28, 30, 32,
    33, 34, 35, 38, **43**

Wanson, M., 13, **21**
Wattal, B.L., 14, **22**
Wedderburn, N., **43**
Wellde, 35, **41**
White, S. Smith-, *see* Smith-
   White, S.
Wijk, H.B. van, *see* van Wijk,
   H.B.
Williams, K., **43**

Wilson, R.J.M., 35, **43**
Woodhill, A.R., 5, 7, 9, 10,
   11, **23**
Wright, C.A., 55, 58, 66,
   69, 71, 72, 74, 76, 77,
   80, 82, 83, **84, 86**

Yen, J.H., 11, **24**

Yoeli, 31, 34, 37, 38; 30,
   42, 43, 44
Yohannes, T.-M. Tesfa-, *see*
   Tesfa-Yohannes, T.-M.
Yu, P., 95, 98, **103**

Zielke, E., 14, **24**

SUBJECT INDEX

Acid phosphatases, hybrid schistosomes, 77

Aedes aegypti, genetic susceptibility, 13-14, 18-19
  irradiated translocations, 17

Aedes cooki, hybridization experiments, 6, 9
  interspecific crossing relationships, 8

Aedes hebrideus, hybridization experiments, 9
  interspecific crossing relationships, 8

Aedes katherinensis, hybridization experiments, 7
  interspecific crossing relationships, 8

Aedes malayensis, hybridization experiments, 5, 7, 9

Aedes pernotatus, hybridization experiments, 9
  interspecific crossing relationships, 8

Aedes polynesiensis, geographical distribution, 1
  hybridization experiments, 5-9
  interspecific crossing relationships, 8

Aedes pseudoscutellaris, hybridization experiments, 5, 7
  interspecific crossing relationship, 8

Aedes scutellaris complex, cytoplasmic incompatibility, 10-12
  genetic susceptibility, 15-16

geographical distribution, 1, 4
  with chromosomal translocations, 16-17, 17-18
  with genes for filarial infection resistance, 18-19

Aedes scutellaris, hybridization experiments, 6, 7, 9
  'Tahafi' form, interspecific crossing relationships, 8

Aedes tabu, hybridization experiments, 6, 9
  interspecific crossing experiments, 8

4-Aminoquinolines, *Plasmodium* resistance, 29

Ampicillin, and cytoplasmic incompatibility, 12

Antibiotics, and cytoplasmic incompatibility, 11-12

Antifolates, *Plasmodium* resistance, 29-30

Biomphalaria, and schistosome hybridization, 67

Biomphalaria glabrata, 68
  and *S. mansoni*, host-parasite relationship, genetics, 45-54
  selection of sub-strains, 47, 48-51
  results, 51-52

Biomphalaria africanus, 68

Biomphalaria alexandrina, 68

Biomphalaria camerunensis, 83

Biomphalaria crystallinus, 69

Biomphalaria forskali group, 69, 70, 71

Biomphalaria pfeifferi, 68

Biomphalaria reticulatus, 67

Biomphalaria rohlfsi, 82, 83

Biomphalaria sudanica, 68

Biomphalaria truncatus, 69, 70, 71

Biomphalaria wrighti, 70, 71

Brugia malayi, mosquito susceptibility, 12
  in *Aedes aegypti*, 13-14

Brugia pahangi, mosquito susceptibility, genetics, 12
  in *Aedes aegypti*, 13-14
  in *Culex pipiens* complex 14-15

Bulinus, and schistosome hybridization, 67-72

Chloramphenicol, and cytoplasmic incompatibility, 12

Chloroquine, *Plasmodium* resistance, 29

Cloning, *Plasmodium*, 26-27
  characteristics, *P. chabaudi*, 34
  P. y. yoelii, 36, 39

Culex pipiens complex, 2
  cytoplasmic incompatibility, 10-12, 16-17
  genetics, 14-15
  and translocation, 17-18

Culex pipiens fatigans, chromosomal translocations, 16-17
  cytoplasmic incompatibility, 16

Dirofilaria immitis, mosquito susceptibility to, 12
Dirofilaria repens, mosquito susceptibility to, 12
Drug-resistance, *Plasmodium* sp., 29-30

Egg morphology, *Schistosoma,* 59-67
Enzyme, patterns, and *Plasmodium* virulence, 39
polymorphism, in *P. berghei* and *P. yoelii,* 28-29
Erythromycin, and cytoplasmic incompatibility, 12

Fasciola hepatica, 81
Filaria, infections, and mosquito genetics, 1-24

Genetic factors, host-parasite relationships, ecology, 87-101
influence, 35-40
malaria parasites, 25-43
neutralist school, 87
recombination experiments, 31-35
selectionist school, 87
techniques, 26-31
mosquito and filarial infections, 1-24, 25-43
Glucose phosphate isomerase (GPI) in cross-fertilization, 32, 33
Plasmodium sp., 29
strain-specific immunity, 35-36

Host-parasite relationships, antigen sharing, 92
genetics, 25-44, 87-101
B. glabrata and *S. mansoni,* 45-54
genotype/phenotype relations, 91
hypotheses, 88-90
models, 94-100
mortality, 94
neutralists, 87
numbers, 93
parasite resistance, 90-91

phenotype variation, 91
Plasmodium, 25-44, 87-101
recombination experiments, 31-35
strain-specific immunity, 35-36
techniques, 26-31
virulence, 36-40
protein polymorphism, 93
selectionists, 87
Hybridization experiments, *Aedes* sp., 3-9
Plasmodium, 26-27
recombination experiments, 31-35
Schistosomes, 55-85
behaviour of cercariae, 72
definitive host infectivity, 74-77
egg morphology, 59-67
interspecific pairings, reciprocity, 58-59
isoenzymes, 77-79

Incompatibility, cytoplasmic, ageing in males, 10
Culex pipiens, 10-12, 16-17
female function, 10
with genes for filarial infection resistance, 18-19
with translocations, 17-18
Isoenzymes, hybrid schistosomes, 77

Lactate dehydrogenase (LDH), in cross-fertilization, 33
hybrid schistosomes, 77
Plasmodium sp., 29
Linum usitatissimum, 91

Malaria parasites, *see Plasmodium*
Malate dehydrogenase, hybrid schistosomes, 77
Mayetiola destructor, 91
Melampsora lini, 91
Mosquito genetics and filarial infections, 1-24

see also Aedes, and specific headings

Paramecium, enzyme polymorphism, 28
Parasitaemia, normal, factors changing, 37-38
6-Phosphogluconate dehydrogenase (6PGD), *Plasmodium* sp., 29
Plasmodium, genetic studies, 25-44
choice of species, 25
cloning, 26-27
genetic techniques, 26-31
host-parasite relationships, 35-40
hybridization, 26-27
markers, 28-31
drug resistance, 29-30
enzyme polymorphism, 28-29
recombination experiments, 31-35
Plasmodium berghei, cloning, 28
drug resistance, 30
enzyme variation, 28
synpholia, 34
Plasmodium chabaudi, cloning, 26, 27, 28
cross-fertilization, 33
enzyme variation, 28-29
Plasmodium falciparum, enzyme variation, 28
strain-specific immunity, 35
Plasmodium gallinaceum, 25
drug resistance, 30
genetic studies, recombination experiments, 31-32
Plasmodium knowlesi, 93
Plasmodium praecox, cloning, 27
Plasmodium vinckei, synpholia, 34
Plasmodium yoelii, cloning, 28
cross-fertilization, 32
drug resistance, 30
enzyme variation, 28-29
strain-specific immunity, 35
synpholia, 34

Plasmodium yoelii nigeriensis, strain-specific immunity, 35
virulence, 40
Plasmodium yoelii yoelii, virulence, 38, 39
Proguanil, *Plasmodium* resistance, 29-30
Pyrimethamine, *Plasmodium* resistance, 29, 30
resistance in cross-fertilization, 32, 33
synpholia, 34

Recombination, genetic, *Plasmodium*, 31-35
cross-fertilization, gametes, 32
Rifampicin, and cytoplasmic incompatibility, 12

Schistosomes, hybridization, 55-85
behaviour of cercariae, 72
definitive host infectivity, 74-77
early work, 56-58
egg morphology, 59-67
intermediate host infectivity, 67-72
interspecific pairings, reciprocity, 58-59
isoenzymes, 77-79
Schistosoma bovis and *S. mattheei*, hybridization, 57
definitive host infectivity, 74
intermediate host infectivity, 68
isoenzymes, 77

Schistosoma haematobium, controlled transmission, 83
and *S. bovis*, hybridization, 57
intermediate host infectivity, 68
isoenzymes, 77-79
and *S. intercalatum*, egg morphology, 60-65
hybridization, 58
behaviour of cercariae, 72, 73-74
definitive host infectivity, 75, 76, 77
focus, 81, 82
influence on taxomony, 80
intermediate host infectivity, 69, 70
isoenzymes, 77-79
and *S. mansoni*, hybridization, 57
Schistosoma mansoni, and *B. glabrata*, host-parasite relationships, genetics, 45-54
selection of sub-strains, 47, 48-51
results, 51-52
and *S. bovis*, hybridization, 58
isoenzymes, 77
and *S. japonicum*, hybridization, 58
cercariae behaviour, 72
and *S. mattheei*, hybridization, 57
and *S. rodhaini*, hybridization, 57
and *B. alexandrina*, 68

Schistosoma mattheei, and *S. haematobium*, hybridization, 57, 81
definitive host infectivity, 74
egg morphology, 60
intermediate host infectivity, 68
and *S. intercalatum*, hybridization, 58
intermediate host infectivity, 69
Streptomycin, and cytoplasmic incompatibility, 12
Sulphonamides, *Plasmodium* resistance to, 29
Synpholia, in genetic studies, 34-35

Tetracycline hydrochloride and cytoplasmic incompatibility, 11, 12
Tetrahymena, enzyme polymorphism, 28
Translocations, chromosomal, *Culex pipiens*, 16-17
with *A. aegypti*, 17
with cytoplasmic incompatibility, 17-18
with genes for filarial infection resistance, 18
Triticum, 91

Virulence of *Plasmodium* strains, 36-40

Wuchereria bancrofti, mosquito susceptibility, 12
Aedes aegypti, 13-14
Culex pipiens complex, 14-15